Pain Management Nursing Exam

SECRETS

Study Guide
Your Key to Exam Success

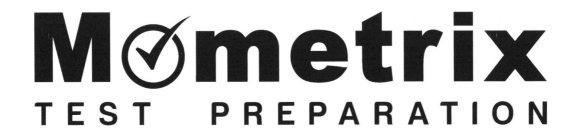

Dear Future Exam Success Story

First of all, **THANK YOU** for purchasing Mometrix study materials!

Second, congratulations! You are one of the few determined test-takers who are committed to doing whatever it takes to excel on your exam. **You have come to the right place.** We developed these study materials with one goal in mind: to deliver you the information you need in a format that's concise and easy to use.

In addition to optimizing your guide for the content of the test, we've outlined our recommended steps for breaking down the preparation process into small, attainable goals so you can make sure you stay on track.

We've also analyzed the entire test-taking process, identifying the most common pitfalls and showing how you can overcome them and be ready for any curveball the test throws you.

Standardized testing is one of the biggest obstacles on your road to success, which only increases the importance of doing well in the high-pressure, high-stakes environment of test day. Your results on this test could have a significant impact on your future, and this guide provides the information and practical advice to help you achieve your full potential on test day.

Your success is our success

We would love to hear from you! If you would like to share the story of your exam success or if you have any questions or comments in regard to our products, please contact us at **800-673-8175** or **support@mometrix.com**.

Thanks again for your business and we wish you continued success!

Sincerely,
The Mometrix Test Preparation Team

Need more help? Check out our flashcards at:
http://mometrixflashcards.com/PainManagement

Copyright © 2020 by Mometrix Media LLC. All rights reserved.
Written and edited by the Mometrix Exam Secrets Test Prep Team
Printed in the United States of America

TABLE OF CONTENTS

INTRODUCTION	1
SECRET KEY #1 – PLAN BIG, STUDY SMALL	2
SECRET KEY #2 – MAKE YOUR STUDYING COUNT	3
SECRET KEY #3 – PRACTICE THE RIGHT WAY	4
SECRET KEY #4 – PACE YOURSELF	6
SECRET KEY #5 – HAVE A PLAN FOR GUESSING	7
TEST-TAKING STRATEGIES	10
FUNDAMENTALS OF PAIN	**15**
SCIENCE OF PAIN	15
PAIN MANAGEMENT MODELS AND THEORIES	17
ETIOLOGY OF PAIN	18
PAIN DIAGNOSES AND SYNDROMES	25
PAIN DESCRIPTORS AND CHARACTERISTICS	27
PAIN HISTORY	28
PAIN ASSESSMENT TECHNIQUES, SCALES, AND TOOLS	33
QUALITY OF LIFE AND FUNCTIONAL ABILITY	41
COPING MECHANISMS AND SUPPORT SYSTEMS	45
POTENTIAL BARRIERS TO PAIN ASSESSMENT	49
RISK ASSESSMENT OF SUBSTANCE USE	50
REASSESSMENT OF PAIN	51
IMPORTANT TERMS	52
INTERVENTIONS	**55**
PLAN OF CARE AND INTERDISCIPLINARY COLLABORATION	55
PHARMACOLOGICAL TREATMENT	56
OPIOID ANALGESICS	58
NON-OPIOID ANALGESICS	61
MEDICATION SAFETY AND MISUSE	65
SIDE EFFECTS OF PHARMACOLOGIC INTERVENTIONS	68
NON-PHARMACOLOGIC PAIN MANAGEMENT	75
IMPORTANT TERMS	81
PROFESSIONAL PRACTICE	**83**
PATIENT, CAREGIVER, AND FAMILY EDUCATION	83
IMPORTANT EDUCATION CONCEPTS	89
EVALUATION OF EDUCATION	90
COMMUNICATION AND CULTURAL CONSIDERATIONS	91
ETHICS	93
DOCUMENTATION REQUIREMENTS	98
STANDARDS OF CARE	100
RESEARCH AND QUALITY IMPROVEMENT	103
IMPORTANT TERMS	106

PAIN MANAGEMENT NURSING PRACTICE TEST	**108**
ANSWER KEY AND EXPLANATIONS	**132**
HOW TO OVERCOME TEST ANXIETY	**153**
CAUSES OF TEST ANXIETY	153
ELEMENTS OF TEST ANXIETY	154
EFFECTS OF TEST ANXIETY	154
PHYSICAL STEPS FOR BEATING TEST ANXIETY	155
MENTAL STEPS FOR BEATING TEST ANXIETY	156
STUDY STRATEGY	157
TEST TIPS	159
IMPORTANT QUALIFICATION	160
THANK YOU	**161**
ADDITIONAL BONUS MATERIAL	**162**

Introduction

Thank you for purchasing this resource! You have made the choice to prepare yourself for a test that could have a huge impact on your future, and this guide is designed to help you be fully ready for test day. Obviously, it's important to have a solid understanding of the test material, but you also need to be prepared for the unique environment and stressors of the test, so that you can perform to the best of your abilities.

For this purpose, the first section that appears in this guide is the **Secret Keys**. We've devoted countless hours to meticulously researching what works and what doesn't, and we've boiled down our findings to the five most impactful steps you can take to improve your performance on the test. We start at the beginning with study planning and move through the preparation process, all the way to the testing strategies that will help you get the most out of what you know when you're finally sitting in front of the test.

We recommend that you start preparing for your test as far in advance as possible. However, if you've bought this guide as a last-minute study resource and only have a few days before your test, we recommend that you skip over the first two Secret Keys since they address a long-term study plan.

If you struggle with **test anxiety**, we strongly encourage you to check out our recommendations for how you can overcome it. Test anxiety is a formidable foe, but it can be beaten, and we want to make sure you have the tools you need to defeat it.

Secret Key #1 – Plan Big, Study Small

There's a lot riding on your performance. If you want to ace this test, you're going to need to keep your skills sharp and the material fresh in your mind. You need a plan that lets you review everything you need to know while still fitting in your schedule. We'll break this strategy down into three categories.

Information Organization

Start with the information you already have: the official test outline. From this, you can make a complete list of all the concepts you need to cover before the test. Organize these concepts into groups that can be studied together, and create a list of any related vocabulary you need to learn so you can brush up on any difficult terms. You'll want to keep this vocabulary list handy once you actually start studying since you may need to add to it along the way.

Time Management

Once you have your set of study concepts, decide how to spread them out over the time you have left before the test. Break your study plan into small, clear goals so you have a manageable task for each day and know exactly what you're doing. Then just focus on one small step at a time. When you manage your time this way, you don't need to spend hours at a time studying. Studying a small block of content for a short period each day helps you retain information better and avoid stressing over how much you have left to do. You can relax knowing that you have a plan to cover everything in time. In order for this strategy to be effective though, you have to start studying early and stick to your schedule. Avoid the exhaustion and futility that comes from last-minute cramming!

Study Environment

The environment you study in has a big impact on your learning. Studying in a coffee shop, while probably more enjoyable, is not likely to be as fruitful as studying in a quiet room. It's important to keep distractions to a minimum. You're only planning to study for a short block of time, so make the most of it. Don't pause to check your phone or get up to find a snack. It's also important to **avoid multitasking**. Research has consistently shown that multitasking will make your studying dramatically less effective. Your study area should also be comfortable and well-lit so you don't have the distraction of straining your eyes or sitting on an uncomfortable chair.

The time of day you study is also important. You want to be rested and alert. Don't wait until just before bedtime. Study when you'll be most likely to comprehend and remember. Even better, if you know what time of day your test will be, set that time aside for study. That way your brain will be used to working on that subject at that specific time and you'll have a better chance of recalling information.

Finally, it can be helpful to team up with others who are studying for the same test. Your actual studying should be done in as isolated an environment as possible, but the work of organizing the information and setting up the study plan can be divided up. In between study sessions, you can discuss with your teammates the concepts that you're all studying and quiz each other on the details. Just be sure that your teammates are as serious about the test as you are. If you find that your study time is being replaced with social time, you might need to find a new team.

Secret Key #2 – Make Your Studying Count

You're devoting a lot of time and effort to preparing for this test, so you want to be absolutely certain it will pay off. This means doing more than just reading the content and hoping you can remember it on test day. It's important to make every minute of study count. There are two main areas you can focus on to make your studying count:

Retention

It doesn't matter how much time you study if you can't remember the material. You need to make sure you are retaining the concepts. To check your retention of the information you're learning, try recalling it at later times with minimal prompting. Try carrying around flashcards and glance at one or two from time to time or ask a friend who's also studying for the test to quiz you.

To enhance your retention, look for ways to put the information into practice so that you can apply it rather than simply recalling it. If you're using the information in practical ways, it will be much easier to remember. Similarly, it helps to solidify a concept in your mind if you're not only reading it to yourself but also explaining it to someone else. Ask a friend to let you teach them about a concept you're a little shaky on (or speak aloud to an imaginary audience if necessary). As you try to summarize, define, give examples, and answer your friend's questions, you'll understand the concepts better and they will stay with you longer. Finally, step back for a big picture view and ask yourself how each piece of information fits with the whole subject. When you link the different concepts together and see them working together as a whole, it's easier to remember the individual components.

Finally, practice showing your work on any multi-step problems, even if you're just studying. Writing out each step you take to solve a problem will help solidify the process in your mind, and you'll be more likely to remember it during the test.

Modality

Modality simply refers to the means or method by which you study. Choosing a study modality that fits your own individual learning style is crucial. No two people learn best in exactly the same way, so it's important to know your strengths and use them to your advantage.

For example, if you learn best by visualization, focus on visualizing a concept in your mind and draw an image or a diagram. Try color-coding your notes, illustrating them, or creating symbols that will trigger your mind to recall a learned concept. If you learn best by hearing or discussing information, find a study partner who learns the same way or read aloud to yourself. Think about how to put the information in your own words. Imagine that you are giving a lecture on the topic and record yourself so you can listen to it later.

For any learning style, flashcards can be helpful. Organize the information so you can take advantage of spare moments to review. Underline key words or phrases. Use different colors for different categories. Mnemonic devices (such as creating a short list in which every item starts with the same letter) can also help with retention. Find what works best for you and use it to store the information in your mind most effectively and easily.

Secret Key #3 – Practice the Right Way

Your success on test day depends not only on how many hours you put into preparing, but also on whether you prepared the right way. It's good to check along the way to see if your studying is paying off. One of the most effective ways to do this is by taking practice tests to evaluate your progress. Practice tests are useful because they show exactly where you need to improve. Every time you take a practice test, pay special attention to these three groups of questions:

- The questions you got wrong
- The questions you had to guess on, even if you guessed right
- The questions you found difficult or slow to work through

This will show you exactly what your weak areas are, and where you need to devote more study time. Ask yourself why each of these questions gave you trouble. Was it because you didn't understand the material? Was it because you didn't remember the vocabulary? Do you need more repetitions on this type of question to build speed and confidence? Dig into those questions and figure out how you can strengthen your weak areas as you go back to review the material.

Additionally, many practice tests have a section explaining the answer choices. It can be tempting to read the explanation and think that you now have a good understanding of the concept. However, an explanation likely only covers part of the question's broader context. Even if the explanation makes sense, **go back and investigate** every concept related to the question until you're positive you have a thorough understanding.

As you go along, keep in mind that the practice test is just that: practice. Memorizing these questions and answers will not be very helpful on the actual test because it is unlikely to have any of the same exact questions. If you only know the right answers to the sample questions, you won't be prepared for the real thing. **Study the concepts** until you understand them fully, and then you'll be able to answer any question that shows up on the test.

It's important to wait on the practice tests until you're ready. If you take a test on your first day of study, you may be overwhelmed by the amount of material covered and how much you need to learn. Work up to it gradually.

On test day, you'll need to be prepared for answering questions, managing your time, and using the test-taking strategies you've learned. It's a lot to balance, like a mental marathon that will have a big impact on your future. Like training for a marathon, you'll need to start slowly and work your way up. When test day arrives, you'll be ready.

Start with the strategies you've read in the first two Secret Keys—plan your course and study in the way that works best for you. If you have time, consider using multiple study resources to get different approaches to the same concepts. It can be helpful to see difficult concepts from more than one angle. Then find a good source for practice tests. Many times, the test website will suggest potential study resources or provide sample tests.

Practice Test Strategy

If you're able to find at least three practice tests, we recommend this strategy:

Untimed and Open-Book Practice

Take the first test with no time constraints and with your notes and study guide handy. Take your time and focus on applying the strategies you've learned.

Timed and Open-Book Practice

Take the second practice test open-book as well, but set a timer and practice pacing yourself to finish in time.

Timed and Closed-Book Practice

Take any other practice tests as if it were test day. Set a timer and put away your study materials. Sit at a table or desk in a quiet room, imagine yourself at the testing center, and answer questions as quickly and accurately as possible.

Keep repeating timed and closed-book tests on a regular basis until you run out of practice tests or it's time for the actual test. Your mind will be ready for the schedule and stress of test day, and you'll be able to focus on recalling the material you've learned.

Secret Key #4 – Pace Yourself

Once you're fully prepared for the material on the test, your biggest challenge on test day will be managing your time. Just knowing that the clock is ticking can make you panic even if you have plenty of time left. Work on pacing yourself so you can build confidence against the time constraints of the exam. Pacing is a difficult skill to master, especially in a high-pressure environment, so **practice is vital**.

Set time expectations for your pace based on how much time is available. For example, if a section has 60 questions and the time limit is 30 minutes, you know you have to average 30 seconds or less per question in order to answer them all. Although 30 seconds is the hard limit, set 25 seconds per question as your goal, so you reserve extra time to spend on harder questions. When you budget extra time for the harder questions, you no longer have any reason to stress when those questions take longer to answer.

Don't let this time expectation distract you from working through the test at a calm, steady pace, but keep it in mind so you don't spend too much time on any one question. Recognize that taking extra time on one question you don't understand may keep you from answering two that you do understand later in the test. If your time limit for a question is up and you're still not sure of the answer, mark it and move on, and come back to it later if the time and the test format allow. If the testing format doesn't allow you to return to earlier questions, just make an educated guess; then put it out of your mind and move on.

On the easier questions, be careful not to rush. It may seem wise to hurry through them so you have more time for the challenging ones, but it's not worth missing one if you know the concept and just didn't take the time to read the question fully. Work efficiently but make sure you understand the question and have looked at all of the answer choices, since more than one may seem right at first.

Even if you're paying attention to the time, you may find yourself a little behind at some point. You should speed up to get back on track, but do so wisely. Don't panic; just take a few seconds less on each question until you're caught up. Don't guess without thinking, but do look through the answer choices and eliminate any you know are wrong. If you can get down to two choices, it is often worthwhile to guess from those. Once you've chosen an answer, move on and don't dwell on any that you skipped or had to hurry through. If a question was taking too long, chances are it was one of the harder ones, so you weren't as likely to get it right anyway.

On the other hand, if you find yourself getting ahead of schedule, it may be beneficial to slow down a little. The more quickly you work, the more likely you are to make a careless mistake that will affect your score. You've budgeted time for each question, so don't be afraid to spend that time. Practice an efficient but careful pace to get the most out of the time you have.

Secret Key #5 – Have a Plan for Guessing

When you're taking the test, you may find yourself stuck on a question. Some of the answer choices seem better than others, but you don't see the one answer choice that is obviously correct. What do you do?

The scenario described above is very common, yet most test takers have not effectively prepared for it. Developing and practicing a plan for guessing may be one of the single most effective uses of your time as you get ready for the exam.

In developing your plan for guessing, there are three questions to address:

- When should you start the guessing process?
- How should you narrow down the choices?
- Which answer should you choose?

When to Start the Guessing Process

Unless your plan for guessing is to select C every time (which, despite its merits, is not what we recommend), you need to leave yourself enough time to apply your answer elimination strategies. Since you have a limited amount of time for each question, that means that if you're going to give yourself the best shot at guessing correctly, you have to decide quickly whether or not you will guess.

Of course, the best-case scenario is that you don't have to guess at all, so first, see if you can answer the question based on your knowledge of the subject and basic reasoning skills. Focus on the key words in the question and try to jog your memory of related topics. Give yourself a chance to bring the knowledge to mind, but once you realize that you don't have (or you can't access) the knowledge you need to answer the question, it's time to start the guessing process.

It's almost always better to start the guessing process too early than too late. It only takes a few seconds to remember something and answer the question from knowledge. Carefully eliminating wrong answer choices takes longer. Plus, going through the process of eliminating answer choices can actually help jog your memory.

Summary: Start the guessing process as soon as you decide that you can't answer the question based on your knowledge.

How to Narrow Down the Choices

The next chapter in this book (**Test-Taking Strategies**) includes a wide range of strategies for how to approach questions and how to look for answer choices to eliminate. You will definitely want to read those carefully, practice them, and figure out which ones work best for you. Here though, we're going to address a mindset rather than a particular strategy.

Your chances of guessing an answer correctly depend on how many options you are choosing from.

How many choices you have	How likely you are to guess correctly
5	20%
4	25%
3	33%
2	50%
1	100%

You can see from this chart just how valuable it is to be able to eliminate incorrect answers and make an educated guess, but there are two things that many test takers do that cause them to miss out on the benefits of guessing:

- Accidentally eliminating the correct answer
- Selecting an answer based on an impression

We'll look at the first one here, and the second one in the next section.

To avoid accidentally eliminating the correct answer, we recommend a thought exercise called **the $5 challenge**. In this challenge, you only eliminate an answer choice from contention if you are willing to bet $5 on it being wrong. Why $5? Five dollars is a small but not insignificant amount of money. It's an amount you could afford to lose but wouldn't want to throw away. And while losing $5 once might not hurt too much, doing it twenty times will set you back $100. In the same way, each small decision you make—eliminating a choice here, guessing on a question there—won't by itself impact your score very much, but when you put them all together, they can make a big difference. By holding each answer choice elimination decision to a higher standard, you can reduce the risk of accidentally eliminating the correct answer.

The $5 challenge can also be applied in a positive sense: If you are willing to bet $5 that an answer choice *is* correct, go ahead and mark it as correct.

Summary: Only eliminate an answer choice if you are willing to bet $5 that it is wrong.

Which Answer to Choose

You're taking the test. You've run into a hard question and decided you'll have to guess. You've eliminated all the answer choices you're willing to bet $5 on. Now you have to pick an answer. Why do we even need to talk about this? Why can't you just pick whichever one you feel like when the time comes?

The answer to these questions is that if you don't come into the test with a plan, you'll rely on your impression to select an answer choice, and if you do that, you risk falling into a trap. The test writers know that everyone who takes their test will be guessing on some of the questions, so they intentionally write wrong answer choices to seem plausible. You still have to pick an answer though, and if the wrong answer choices are designed to look right, how can you ever be sure that you're not falling for their trap? The best solution we've found to this dilemma is to take the decision out of your hands entirely. Here is the process we recommend:

Once you've eliminated any choices that you are confident (willing to bet $5) are wrong, select the first remaining choice as your answer.

Whether you choose to select the first remaining choice, the second, or the last, the important thing is that you use some preselected standard. Using this approach guarantees that you will not be enticed into selecting an answer choice that looks right, because you are not basing your decision on how the answer choices look.

This is not meant to make you question your knowledge. Instead, it is to help you recognize the difference between your knowledge and your impressions. There's a huge difference between thinking an answer is right because of what you know, and thinking an answer is right because it looks or sounds like it should be right.

Summary: To ensure that your selection is appropriately random, make a predetermined selection from among all answer choices you have not eliminated.

Test-Taking Strategies

This section contains a list of test-taking strategies that you may find helpful as you work through the test. By taking what you know and applying logical thought, you can maximize your chances of answering any question correctly!

It is very important to realize that every question is different and every person is different: no single strategy will work on every question, and no single strategy will work for every person. That's why we've included all of them here, so you can try them out and determine which ones work best for different types of questions and which ones work best for you.

Question Strategies

READ CAREFULLY

Read the question and answer choices carefully. Don't miss the question because you misread the terms. You have plenty of time to read each question thoroughly and make sure you understand what is being asked. Yet a happy medium must be attained, so don't waste too much time. You must read carefully, but efficiently.

CONTEXTUAL CLUES

Look for contextual clues. If the question includes a word you are not familiar with, look at the immediate context for some indication of what the word might mean. Contextual clues can often give you all the information you need to decipher the meaning of an unfamiliar word. Even if you can't determine the meaning, you may be able to narrow down the possibilities enough to make a solid guess at the answer to the question.

PREFIXES

If you're having trouble with a word in the question or answer choices, try dissecting it. Take advantage of every clue that the word might include. Prefixes and suffixes can be a huge help. Usually they allow you to determine a basic meaning. Pre- means before, post- means after, pro - is positive, de- is negative. From prefixes and suffixes, you can get an idea of the general meaning of the word and try to put it into context.

HEDGE WORDS

Watch out for critical hedge words, such as *likely, may, can, sometimes, often, almost, mostly, usually, generally, rarely,* and *sometimes*. Question writers insert these hedge phrases to cover every possibility. Often an answer choice will be wrong simply because it leaves no room for exception. Be on guard for answer choices that have definitive words such as *exactly* and *always*.

SWITCHBACK WORDS

Stay alert for *switchbacks*. These are the words and phrases frequently used to alert you to shifts in thought. The most common switchback words are *but, although,* and *however*. Others include *nevertheless, on the other hand, even though, while, in spite of, despite, regardless of.* Switchback words are important to catch because they can change the direction of the question or an answer choice.

Face Value

When in doubt, use common sense. Accept the situation in the problem at face value. Don't read too much into it. These problems will not require you to make wild assumptions. If you have to go beyond creativity and warp time or space in order to have an answer choice fit the question, then you should move on and consider the other answer choices. These are normal problems rooted in reality. The applicable relationship or explanation may not be readily apparent, but it is there for you to figure out. Use your common sense to interpret anything that isn't clear.

Answer Choice Strategies

Answer Selection

The most thorough way to pick an answer choice is to identify and eliminate wrong answers until only one is left, then confirm it is the correct answer. Sometimes an answer choice may immediately seem right, but be careful. The test writers will usually put more than one reasonable answer choice on each question, so take a second to read all of them and make sure that the other choices are not equally obvious. As long as you have time left, it is better to read every answer choice than to pick the first one that looks right without checking the others.

Answer Choice Families

An answer choice family consists of two (in rare cases, three) answer choices that are very similar in construction and cannot all be true at the same time. If you see two answer choices that are direct opposites or parallels, one of them is usually the correct answer. For instance, if one answer choice says that quantity x increases and another either says that quantity x decreases (opposite) or says that quantity y increases (parallel), then those answer choices would fall into the same family. An answer choice that doesn't match the construction of the answer choice family is more likely to be incorrect. Most questions will not have answer choice families, but when they do appear, you should be prepared to recognize them.

Eliminate Answers

Eliminate answer choices as soon as you realize they are wrong, but make sure you consider all possibilities. If you are eliminating answer choices and realize that the last one you are left with is also wrong, don't panic. Start over and consider each choice again. There may be something you missed the first time that you will realize on the second pass.

Avoid Fact Traps

Don't be distracted by an answer choice that is factually true but doesn't answer the question. You are looking for the choice that answers the question. Stay focused on what the question is asking for so you don't accidentally pick an answer that is true but incorrect. Always go back to the question and make sure the answer choice you've selected actually answers the question and is not merely a true statement.

Extreme Statements

In general, you should avoid answers that put forth extreme actions as standard practice or proclaim controversial ideas as established fact. An answer choice that states the "process should be used in certain situations, if…" is much more likely to be correct than one that states the "process should be discontinued completely." The first is a calm rational statement and doesn't even make a definitive, uncompromising stance, using a hedge word *if* to provide wiggle room, whereas the second choice is a radical idea and far more extreme.

BENCHMARK

As you read through the answer choices and you come across one that seems to answer the question well, mentally select that answer choice. This is not your final answer, but it's the one that will help you evaluate the other answer choices. The one that you selected is your benchmark or standard for judging each of the other answer choices. Every other answer choice must be compared to your benchmark. That choice is correct until proven otherwise by another answer choice beating it. If you find a better answer, then that one becomes your new benchmark. Once you've decided that no other choice answers the question as well as your benchmark, you have your final answer.

PREDICT THE ANSWER

Before you even start looking at the answer choices, it is often best to try to predict the answer. When you come up with the answer on your own, it is easier to avoid distractions and traps because you will know exactly what to look for. The right answer choice is unlikely to be word-for-word what you came up with, but it should be a close match. Even if you are confident that you have the right answer, you should still take the time to read each option before moving on.

General Strategies

TOUGH QUESTIONS

If you are stumped on a problem or it appears too hard or too difficult, don't waste time. Move on! Remember though, if you can quickly check for obviously incorrect answer choices, your chances of guessing correctly are greatly improved. Before you completely give up, at least try to knock out a couple of possible answers. Eliminate what you can and then guess at the remaining answer choices before moving on.

CHECK YOUR WORK

Since you will probably not know every term listed and the answer to every question, it is important that you get credit for the ones that you do know. Don't miss any questions through careless mistakes. If at all possible, try to take a second to look back over your answer selection and make sure you've selected the correct answer choice and haven't made a costly careless mistake (such as marking an answer choice that you didn't mean to mark). This quick double check should more than pay for itself in caught mistakes for the time it costs.

PACE YOURSELF

It's easy to be overwhelmed when you're looking at a page full of questions; your mind is confused and full of random thoughts, and the clock is ticking down faster than you would like. Calm down and maintain the pace that you have set for yourself. Especially as you get down to the last few minutes of the test, don't let the small numbers on the clock make you panic. As long as you are on track by monitoring your pace, you are guaranteed to have time for each question.

DON'T RUSH

It is very easy to make errors when you are in a hurry. Maintaining a fast pace in answering questions is pointless if it makes you miss questions that you would have gotten right otherwise. Test writers like to include distracting information and wrong answers that seem right. Taking a little extra time to avoid careless mistakes can make all the difference in your test score. Find a pace that allows you to be confident in the answers that you select.

Keep Moving

Panicking will not help you pass the test, so do your best to stay calm and keep moving. Taking deep breaths and going through the answer elimination steps you practiced can help to break through a stress barrier and keep your pace.

Final Notes

The combination of a solid foundation of content knowledge and the confidence that comes from practicing your plan for applying that knowledge is the key to maximizing your performance on test day. As your foundation of content knowledge is built up and strengthened, you'll find that the strategies included in this chapter become more and more effective in helping you quickly sift through the distractions and traps of the test to isolate the correct answer.

Now it's time to move on to the test content chapters of this book, but be sure to keep your goal in mind. As you read, think about how you will be able to apply this information on the test. If you've already seen sample questions for the test and you have an idea of the question format and style, try to come up with questions of your own that you can answer based on what you're reading. This will give you valuable practice applying your knowledge in the same ways you can expect to on test day.

Good luck and good studying!

Fundamentals of Pain

Science of Pain

NOCICEPTIVE PAIN

Pain arises from the stimulation of pain receptors within the body. Noxious stimuli such as extreme pressure, heat, cold, or mechanical tissue damage will signal the body of the need for correction and protection through the sensation of pain. Pain of this nature is referred to as **"nociceptive" pain.** It is detected by specialized nerve endings known as nociceptors. When noxious stimuli are detected by the nociceptors, they are activated or sensitized, causing the transduction of the noxious stimuli into electrochemical impulses. These electrochemical impulses are sent to the spinal cord and the central nervous system, delivering the message of pain. A reflexive and/or cognitive response is the result.

The two types of nociceptive pain include:

- Somatic pain
- Visceral pain

SOMATIC PAIN

Nociceptive pain is subdivided into somatic and visceral pain. These two types of nociceptive pain can be identified by the quality of pain and their unique clinical presentations. **Somatic pain** is caused by nociceptors found in cutaneous and subcutaneous tissues, bone, periarticular soft tissues, joints, and muscles being excited and sensitized by painful (noxious) stimuli. Pain sensations are ultimately received by the brain. Topographically, somatic pain is usually well localized. It can be sporadic or constant, and may be described by the patient with words like "aching, stabbing, gnawing and/or throbbing." Somatic pain has four physiological processes involved in its production and sensation. They are: transduction, transmission, modulation and perception.

VISCERAL PAIN

Visceral pain is a subdivision of nociceptive pain. The neural pathways of visceral pain are less sensorially definitive than those of somatic pain, thus visceral pain is more difficult to accurately localize. Visceral pain can be described as either intermittent or constant, and is diffuse in nature. People may describe visceral pain as "dull, colicky or squeezing" sensations. Other nociceptive visceral pain facts and features include:

- Not all visceral organs can induce pain. The liver, kidney, lung parenchyma and most solid viscera are not susceptible to pain. However, adjacent tissues may be quite sensitive (such as the kidney's ureters, when encountering kidney stones, the bronchi of the lungs, or the gall bladder underlying the liver, etc.).
- Visceral pain is not always linked to an injury of the viscera.
- Visceral pain is poorly localized and diffuse.
- Pain can be "referent" in nature, i.e., manifest well away from the actual site of the painful stimulus.
- Visceral pain is also escorted by autonomic and motor responses.

Non-Nociceptive Pain

Non-nociceptive pain is divided into two subsets: neuropathic and idiopathic. **Neuropathic pain** is a result of injury to the peripheral or central nervous system's neural structures. This type of pain is thought to be maintained by abnormal somatosensory processing in the periphery or central nervous system. Patients use words like "sharp or burning" when describing neuropathic pain. **Idiopathic pain** (sometimes termed psychogenic pain) describes a vast collection of poorly understood pain states. With some patients, no physiologic problem can be named as the causative factor. For others, the pain and symptoms are largely out of proportion to the underlying pathology. Myofascial pain syndrome is one example of idiopathic pain.

Neuropathic Pain

Neuropathic pain is not completely understood. It appears that previously normal nerve fibers may become damaged, injured, or dysfunctional as a result of the effects of diabetes, multiple sclerosis, shingles, or other such pathology. Inaccurate signals of pain may then be transmitted. A theory surrounding injury-induced neuropathic pain postulates that the sensitizing mechanism activated by acute pain may become disordered by injury. When the neural tissue undergoes constant assault from sensory neurons in the spinal cord, including pain signals from the periphery, the neurons may become oversensitive to all messages coming in (including non-noxious stimuli). The pain pathway is then ardent continuously. This process is normal with an acute injury, but when it doesn't wane with healing, it is then considered diseased.

- **Central neuropathic pain** is neuropathic pain that begins at any point along the central nervous system.
- **Peripheral neuropathic pain** is created at the level of a nerve ending or along the nerve course to the root itself.

Transient (Acute) Pain

Acute pain is of short duration (0-7 days), and announces the presence of a noxious stimulus that will produce actual tissue damage or has the potential to eventually do damage. Described as mild to severe, acute pain can be caused by either an unknown or known source. Acute pain is typically a single, treatable occurrence. The sensation of acute pain involves peripheral nociceptors. Occasionally, acute pain is associated with autonomic nervous system responses such as tachycardia, hypertension, sweating and vasoconstriction. Treating acute pain is often urgent and done while the source of the pain is being explored. Occasionally, the process of diagnosing a condition can require temporarily deferring or minimizing pain treatment. There is minimal to mild psychological involvement in acute pain. Acute pain can be classified as: acute, subacute, ongoing acute and recurrent acute.

Persistent (Chronic) Pain

Pain that is not being resolved and is not expected to resolve or pain that is lasting longer than traditional length of resolution can be considered **chronic pain**. There is no definitive timeline for determining chronic pain, however, pain can be considered chronic after about three months.

Chronic nonmalignant pain can be rooted in both unknown and non-life-threatening causes. Treating chronic pain is focused on pain elimination or reduction. Often, patients suffering from chronic pain do not readily respond to conventional pain management treatments. This type of pain can be lifelong.

Chronic malignant pain is caused by cancer-related physiologic processes. The cancer itself, treatment of the cancer, or concurrent disease can all be the origin of chronic malignant pain. This type of pain maybe experienced acutely, chronically or sporadically and is rarely accompanied by a sympathetic nervous system response.

Pain Management Models and Theories

GATE CONTROL THEORY OF PAIN

In 1965, **Melzack and Walls** produced the "gate control" theory of pain by critiquing and reshaping existing theories and data. Components of specificity theory, pattern theory and numerous psychological theories were all included by Melzack and Walls. Through further supporting research and new clinical advances, gate-control theory has gained extensive acceptance and validation. In 1983 and 1996 Melzack and Walls added propositions to the theory based upon new research derived from their original theory. Gate control theory is presently the dominant model of pain theory, although some continue to feel that it poorly addresses chronic pain.

Gate-control theory describes pain as a "complex perceptual experience influenced by physiologic and psychological factors unique to the individual." The **gate control theory of pain** contends that both nociceptive (pain) and non-nociceptive (non-pain) sensations are processed through the dorsal horn of the spinal cord. Afferent nerves (those that bring signals to the spinal cord and brain, rather than relaying commands from the brain to the body) are composed of various diameter fibers. The smaller nociceptive fibers, $A\delta$ and C (transmitting acute and chronic pain signals, respectively), and the larger non-nociceptive fibers ($A\beta$) have the capacity to interfere with each other. Large ($A\beta$) fiber signals tend to shut out or close the pain gate, while small fiber signals tend to open it (with the gate "swinging" open or closed in deference to the more predominant signal flows). Thus, where non-nociceptive fiber signals predominate, nociceptive signals may be occluded, thereby reducing the sensation of pain. This theory helps explain why non-nociceptive stimuli such as massage and TENS (transcutaneous electrical stimulation) treatments are able to reduce otherwise very painful sensations.

ACTION SYSTEM AND T CELLS

Peripheral afferent nerve signals are brought into the spinal cord via **spinal "T" (transmission) cells,** and modulated by spinal gating in the dorsal horn. When T cell transmission of noxious stimuli reaches a critical level, the **"action system"** is activated. The action system incorporates the motivational-affective and sensory-discriminatory systems that both interact with the central control processes of the brain. These three systems then engage the motor system to determine how the body will react. Thus, the action system directly correlates the behaviors of pain with pain intensity.

Melzack and Wall concluded in 1983 that, despite extensive research, the T cells do not appear to be contained in one single, localized structure. Instead, a theory was proposed that the T cells are integral to the action system, participating in a complex process of communications between multilayered neuromatrices.

EFFECTS OF NERVE IMPULSES ON THE GATING MECHANISM IN THE DORSAL HORN

Melzack and Wall initially theorized that a specialized system, the **central intensity monitor**, made up of components from the motivational-affective, limbic and reticular structures helped to control the proposed gating system. Largely, they felt, this was moderated by the central control process of the brain. Further, they theorized that the central control process affects the gating mechanism of the dorsal horn and the discriminative and motivational systems by evaluating pain based upon conditions of past experience. Later, however, it was found that unconscious central control processes and conscious motivational-affective structures have a greater role in the perception of pain intensity than had been previously recognized.

INTENSITY AND SPECIFICITY THEORIES OF PAIN

The **intensity theory** of pain has its inception in the 4th century BC, beginning with foundational concepts presented by Plato, that were built upon by many theorists thereafter. Plato originally posited that pain is actually an emotional response or experience to overstimulation of the sensation of touch. The intensity of the stimulation dictates the amount of pain experienced. In this theory, intensity refers to the sum of sensations of touch over a period of time.

The **specificity theory**, presented by Von Frey in 1895 but a composite of various theorists preceding him, is considered one of the earliest modern theories attempting to describe pain. More biological/physiological than emotional in nature, the specificity theory proposes that there are specific pain receptors that sense a painful stimulus and then send a pain signal to a part of the brain is referred to as the "pain center." This pain center is considered a separate and specific entity, such as those that are dedicated towards sight or sound. Von Frey referenced the sensations of heat and cold to exemplify the specificity of these pain receptors, noting that pain receptors function separately but similarly to these temperature receptors.

PATTERN THEORY OF PAIN

The **pattern theory** of pain disregarded the thoughts specific to the intensity and specificity theories of pain. It does not separate the systems/receptors of pain and rather puts forth that pain receptors are shared with other receptors of sensation (such as touch). These receptors are able to differentiate the pattern of dangerous/damaging sensations from those that are not, based on the pattern of the sensation. When certain damaging patterns are detected that result from high intensity touch, temperature, etc., those patterns are then separated from non-painful sensations and then sent to the brain. The brain (nervous system) then responds accordingly.

Etiology of Pain

CAUSES OF PAIN IN CANCER PATIENTS

Four **causes of pain that a cancer patient may struggle with** include the following:

1. **Pain directly related to the cancer**: Cancer patients may suffer from nociceptive pain when a tumor or mass invades, stretches or pushes on a pain-sensitive part of the body. This is the most common type of pain a cancer patient experiences.
2. **Pain indirectly related to cancer**: As cancer advances and becomes debilitating, tissue damage (pressure sores, muscle and joint pain from immobility and muscle wasting, etc.) will often cause significant pain.
3. **Incidental pain**: Cancer patients can also suffer from pain that is unrelated to their cancer. Most cancer patients are elderly and may already be afflicted with other degenerative conditions that cause pain (osteoarthritis, etc.). These pain sources should be treated as promptly and vigorously as the cancer-related pain.
4. **Treatment-related pain**: Many, if not most, of the treatments available for cancer can and will cause varying degrees of pain.

BONE PAIN RELATED TO CANCER AND CANCER METASTASES

Metastatic cancer of the breast, lung, prostate, and thyroid, and multiple myeloma, are the most common types of cancer to metastasize to the bone. **Bone tumors** are the most prevalent cause of cancer pain. Because this type of pain is somatic in nature, unless also involving a pathologic fracture or tumor disruption of a nerve, it is regularly expressed as being focal and constant. However, under certain circumstances the pain can be referred and widespread. Tumors can cause **bone pain** by activating nociceptors through pressure or ischemia, or by secreting algesic (pain producing) substances. The vertebral column, skull, humerus, ribs, pelvis and femur are common sites for bone metastases. Bone pain can also be caused by treatments for cancer. Steroid treatment and radiation both have side effects that can cause bone pain.

Psychological Issues of Cancer Patients Relating to Pain

Cancer patients have **psychological issues** related to their pain that need to be addressed. Fear of pain and fear of dying are two important issues addressed in palliative care. General psychodynamic counseling and cognitive-behavioral counseling help adult cancer patients to cope better with anxiety and depression, and in turn help them to better manage their pain. Becoming familiar with the patient's experiences and attitudes about pain will also help the attending nurse to provide more effective care. Further, McCaffrey's pain definition, "pain is what the patient says it is and exists whenever he or she says it does" will help guide a nurse in assessing and caring for a patient's pain. Psychological aspects of pain cannot be separated from the experience and must always be meaningfully addressed.

Chronic and Acute Lower Back Pain

Chronic lower back pain is defined as any low back pain that lasts longer than seven to twelve weeks. Some practitioners more loosely define chronic lower back pain as any pain that lasts longer than should be expected for the healing process. Acute lower back pain is indicative of a nociceptive response to an injury. All of the structures in the spine have nociceptors, so any injuries will cause pain. Considerable research supports a correlation between lower back pain and general poor health. In particular, essential levels of activity necessary to maintain overall conditioning, cardiovascular function, bowel motility, and other features of physical well-being are substantially reduced. Further, many facets of poor health predispose someone to lower back pain. They include: smoking, obesity, inadequate physical activity, and reduced strength and flexibility.

Relation of Osteoporosis, Osteoarthritis and Spondylolysis to Chronic Back Pain

Osteoporosis is a loss (often severe) in bone density. Deformity, fractures and risk for fractures all increase with osteoporosis. Hips carry the greatest risk of fracture, however, spinal fractures can and do occur. Three symptoms observed in osteoporosis are: spinal deformity, decrease in height and chronic back pain.

Osteoarthritis is inflammatory in nature and is also a common source of chronic back pain. The cervical spine is particularly vulnerable to osteoarthritis. Fractures in this part of the spine are invariably painful, and can also lead to paralysis and death.

A patient presenting with chronic back pain may also be suffering from a fracture of the "pars interarticularis," or neural arch, that is found between the inferior and superior articulating spinal processes or facets. This condition is called **spondylolysis**. Spondylolysis can advance to spondylolisthesis (displacement or misalignment of one vertebra from another). Surgical correction is generally required.

Herniated Intervertebral Disk and Chronic Back Pain

Pain from a **herniated intervertebral disc** is caused by physical pressure placed on the nerve root by a protruding disk. In a healthy back, the disc (which is composed of an inner gelatinous material called the nucleus pulposus, contained inside a fibrous sheath called the annulus fibrosus) rests securely between the vertebra. As the annulus fibrosus ages, it may weaken or tear, and thus does not hold the nucleus pulposus correctly. The herniation, or extrusion, of the nucleus pulposus through the annulus fibrosus puts pressure on the spinal cord and/or the nearby nerves. Chronic pain results, as well as the possibility of neurological symptoms, including but not restricted to: weakness or loss of motor function, weakened or absent deep tendon reflexes, and even loss of sensation to the affected extremity.

ABDOMINAL PAIN

When pain receptors found within **abdominal organs** are activated, visceral pain occurs. Visceral pain can be localized in the abdomen or referred to other places in the body. Interestingly, the abdominal pain sensors do not respond to surgical cutting. They do, however, feel distention, twisting, traction and stretching. Thus, visceral pain is usually poorly localized, making the source of this type of pain difficult to identify. Abdominal pain can be both chronic and acute. Chronic pain is usually defined as pain persisting six months or more, or as pain that persists after healing has occurred. Many patients who experience abdominal pain have also experienced sexual and/or physical abuse, making treatment difficult and often requiring multidisciplinary involvement.

IBS

Irritable bowel syndrome (IBS) is characterized as a functional bowel disorder of unknown origin. Approximately 15% of the population suffers from irritable bowel syndrome. Patients with IBS have a chronic pattern of abdominal-pelvic pain and bowel dysfunction, including both constipation and/or diarrhea. The symptoms may include: pain (both abdominal and pelvic or both), bloating, belching, excessive flatus, diarrhea, constipation, passing mucus, painful defecation and a feeling of incomplete evacuation of the bowel. As with many other painful syndromes, IBS may be accompanied depression and anxiety and is often worse during stressful periods and during the premenstrual phase of a woman's cycle.

MIGRAINE

Migraine is a painful, transiently disabling form of headache.

- **Phase one** of a migraine headache precedes the painful headache attack by hours or even days. A person may experience altered mood, irritability, depression or euphoria, fatigue, yawning, excessive sleepiness, craving for chocolate, and/or other vegetative symptoms.
- **Phase two** is the *aura*. Typical aura symptoms are manifest as visual and/or sensory phenomena, including motor weakness, poor coordination and/or (rarely) dysphasic symptoms like difficulty finding words. Generally, the aura attack occurs before the headache by minutes, although they can occur together. Not all migraine sufferers will experience the aura phase. Patients may describe their aura as visual flashing, jagged lights, double vision, or loss of vision, as well as sensory "pins and needles" prickling on the face or involving the limbs. Some may also experience vertigo.
- The **third migraine phase** is the *headache phase*. The headache is typically unilateral and alternates from side to side with different attacks. Some people will report bilateral pain, with greater intensity on one side. The alternating of pain between sides of the head is a definitive characteristic of migraine headache. The pain is gradual in onset and works toward a peak. Nausea, vomiting and light sensitivity also occur. Movement exacerbates the pain, thus lying down is the more typical relief-seeking behavior.
- **Phase four** of migraine headache is *resolution*. Somnolence and sleeping for one to two hours are the most common natural resolution. Pharmacological intervention is the most effective way to resolve a migraine headache.

- **Phase five** is termed *"postdrome"* and is experienced by 94% of migraine sufferers. This phase lasts about 24 hours, and symptoms may include: feeling drained and exhausted, or a sense of elation and euphoria.

Cluster Headaches

Cluster headache is one of the most debilitating and excruciating of all headache disorders. It is defined by several characteristics:

- Cluster headaches are **extremely painful,** often described as worse than a migraine and worse than childbirth by female patients.
- Cluster headache attacks can occur **up to eight times per day** and are clustered **over a period of weeks to months,** followed by an absence of the attacks for months or even years.
- Cluster headaches **run on a regular schedule.** Patients are often awakened during the night at the exact same time. These headache attacks also have a seasonal dimension, frequently occurring at the same time of year (often fall and spring). Cluster headache always presents on the same side and carries a strong familial tendency.

Symptoms

Cluster headache onset is virtually immediate, with a rapid escalation in severity. It is described as a deep boring or searing pain, often localized in the eye and occasionally in the temple. During a cluster headache attack pain is accompanied by autonomic symptoms such as nasal congestion, eye watering, facial flushing and forehead sweating. Patients with cluster headache tend to writhe in pain, moving, walking, sitting or rocking and are unable to remain still as they search for relief. There are no nausea, vomiting, or visual symptoms like those found with migraines, even though the pain is considerable and is often localized behind the eye. Symptoms are likely to be individualized and specific to each person's attacks. Because cluster headache symptoms are very distinctive, it is relatively easy to diagnose.

Tension-Type Headache

The most common type of headache is **tension-type headache (TTH).** Almost everyone will experience or has already experienced this type of headache. These headaches are less intense than migraine headaches or cluster headaches and are usually resolved with an over-the-counter medication. Tension-type headache is often associated with a sense of pressure or tight band-like aching affecting the whole head. There are no other associated symptoms. However, if these headaches are not treated, they can sometimes progress to migraine-type intensity with the associated symptoms of nausea and light sensitivity. Patients may have tension-type headaches and migraine headaches as well. Patients should be warned against overuse of the medications used to control these headaches. Overuse can lead to analgesic rebound headaches.

General Temporal Mandibular Joint Disorders and Diseases

It is often very difficult to establish an exact cause of masticatory pain. Taking a detailed history is usually essential to securing a proper diagnosis. These disorders are widespread and classified in many different ways. **TMJ (temporomandibular joint disorder or masticatory muscle spasm)** is the most common of all masticatory system disorders. It is more common in women than men, and some research shows that 28% to 88% of people have presenting signs of dysfunction although most are unaware. The signs and symptoms are as follows: mandibular motion decrease, impaired masticatory function, pain upon palpation of the muscles or joint. Patients suffering from TMJ may also exhibit one or more of the following symptoms: temporomandibular joint sounds (e.g., popping, cracking, etc.), stiffness and/or fatigue in the jaw, pain when the mouth is opened wide, and locking of the jaw. X-rays are not diagnostic.

TREATMENT OF TMJ

Noninvasive treatment works best for most patients suffering from TMJ. The following are key **noninvasive treatment** elements:

1. **Reassurance** is needed, and it is helpful for patients to realize that the syndrome is very common. Educate patients on the benign characteristic of general muscle spasm and explain how they usually precipitate TMJ themselves.
2. Immobilization of the mandible is not recommended. However, **reduced motion** is helpful. Thus, have patients follow a soft diet for up to two weeks and encourage them to keep their mouth from opening wide (as when yawning or laughing) for that same period of time. Further, no gum chewing, fingernail biting or clenching the jaw, helps as well.
3. Using **heat** on the sides of the face will provide comfort and relieve pain.
4. Success with medicinal intervention can be achieved by using **non-steroidal anti-inflammatory analgesics. Antidepressants** have also been known to produce results in treating chronic pain, including TMJ. There is a strong psychological component to TMJ that antidepressants may treat effectively.

PAIN IN HIV PATIENTS

Research shows pain to be significantly under-treated in the **HIV** population, as well as being under-recognized. Treatment is complicated by the fact that most HIV patients are likely to be on a wide variety of medications (polypharmacy) that may produce interactions with any additional pain medications. Further, diarrhea is a common side effect of HIV (due to medications and opportunistic infections), and it will often interfere with pain drug absorption and thus impede treatment of pain through analgesics. HIV pain is considered to be comparable in intensity to cancer pain. HIV patients however, often experience more than one painful syndrome at a time. It is therefore important to treat acute pain before it converts to chronic pain, and a pain sustaining process begins.

PSYCHOLOGICAL ASPECTS OF TREATING PAIN

Drug abuse and addiction are two risk factors that are important in treating HIV pain. Patients with a history of substance abuse experience pain as intensely and fully as their drug-free counterparts. They are, however, much more likely to be under-treated for pain. This under-treatment occurs for at least two reasons. First, patients in recovery may be reluctant to agree to appropriate opioid therapy. And, second, physicians are often disinclined to prescribe adequate opioid medications out of fear of reengaging or worsening addictive issues. However, pain in HIV is believed to increase as the disease progresses. This also gives HIV pain a greater psychological impact on its sufferers, as it signals further progression of the disease. Using a multidisciplinary approach to treating HIV pain will lead to more successful treatment of HIV pain.

SICKLE CELL DISEASE
ACUTE PAIN IN ADULTS

Pain is a distinguishing feature of **sickle cell disease**. Acute sickle cell pain crises last an average of 10.3 days in adults and cause 90% of sickle cell admissions to the hospital. Patients may describe their pain as coming from the bones, usually involving the arms, hands, legs, feet, or back. Pain in the abdomen or chest may also be reported. The primary mechanism of acute sickle cell pain is actually tissue hypoxia rather than direct tissue or nerve damage. Thus, it is considered to be ischemic pain. Sickle cell precipitated vaso-occlusion causes the ischemia and can produce both visceral and somatic pain. This pain is often highly disruptive to activities of daily living (relationships, employment, and personal care) and should be treated very aggressively.

Chronic Pain in Adults

Chronic pain may develop as acute episodes increase in frequency and intensity. Damage to tissues from the highly destructive vaso-occlusive attacks of acute pain crises bring about chronic injury, leading to chronic pain. Bone infarction causing aseptic necrosis of the hip, as well as vertebral compression fractures and chronic low back pain are examples of chronic pain sources in a patient diagnosed with sickle cell disease. The ischemic attacks caused by sickle cell disease can also produce infarctions in many organs, causing considerable damage and eventually chronic pain. Acute pain crises often occur on top of chronic pain, with acute pain recurring at different frequencies for different patients. The patient's report of pain should be taken as the standard by which the pain is treated.

Treating Pain in Children

A pain crisis due to **sickle cell disease in a child** can last from several hours to weeks. A pain crisis usually produces pain in the extremities, chest, lower back and abdomen. Pain is often managed at home by parents and other caregivers. All caregivers should be educated in the use of opioids, and in avoiding precipitating factors of acute attacks if they are known. Education about a variety of other coping mechanisms can also be useful in pain management and reduction. Children are often under-treated with opioids due to fears of precipitating an addiction. Education on the proper use and management of these drugs will help the child achieve better pain control and greatly reduce the likelihood of future drug dependence. Parents and daily care givers should be given guidelines to follow concerning pain management and when to seek further medical support and help.

Pain During Perinatal Labor and Delivery

Factors

Many **factors influence pain during labor and delivery**, including:

- **Physical factors** such as the size of the baby's head as related to the mother's pelvis, which may have an effect on pain. Different laboring positions can also alter pain, as well as reducing the potential for maternal exhaustion.
- **Physiological and biochemical causes:** Adrenocorticotropic hormones increase as labor progresses as well as plasma endorphins that contribute to reducing pain.
- **Psychological factors:** Pain perception and avoidance behavior is escalated by fear, apprehension, and anxiety. Ignorance and inaccurate information regarding the labor and delivery process can contribute to fear. The nature of the relationship between the new mother and her partner is also strongly correlated with pain perception during labor and delivery.
- **Cultural and ethnic factors:** May influence the process of labor and delivery. Different rituals and beliefs can either increase or diminish pain perception.

Pain Management in Labor

Types of **pain management available to the laboring mother** are:

- **Non-medicinal pain management strategies:** This includes breathing techniques (slow paced breathing, and patterned breathing), conscious relaxation, focal point concentration, massage, and heat and cold therapy. Walking, rocking, coaching support and changing of positions are also successful non-invasive methods to help cope with labor and delivery pain.

- **Pharmacological analgesia:** This includes narcotics (Demerol, Fentanyl, and Nubain) to control labor and delivery pain. However, while the pain will be lessened it will not be entirely gone. Side effects for mother and baby (both in utero and after delivery) differ with each medication and should be fully considered before use. Some of these medications also carry some risk of altering labor, and that should be weighed as well.
- **Regional anesthesia** (i.e., a "saddle block", etc.) provides complete pain control in most cases. However, spotty or unilateral coverage can sometimes be reported. In addition to pain control, other side effects include: blood pressure, body temperature and movement are all compromised. Side effects to the baby and mother should be considered, as well as the slowed labor that often accompanies epidural use. AWHONN (the Association of Women's Health, Obstetric, and Neonatal Nurses) approves the use of epidural and intrathecal therapies, when indicated. The laboring woman should always have the final say in what treatment methods are used, unless she is incapacitated by the process or she and her baby are in jeopardy.

POSTOPERATIVE PAIN

FACTORS DETERMINING INTENSITY, QUALITY, AND DURATION

The **primary factors influencing postoperative pain** include:

- The **site, nature and duration** of the surgery. The incision type used, as well as the amount of trauma inflicted at the surgical site are significant factors.
- The patient's physiological and psychological make up.
- The **preoperative preparation** of the patient in regards to psychological, physical and pharmacological needs.
- Serious related postoperative **complications.**
- Tolerance and management of **anesthesia.**
- The **quality** of postoperative care.

Unfortunately, research shows that some inadequate analgesic control of postoperative pain is due to nurses possessing an inadequate or inaccurate understanding of narcotics pharmacology. Poor pharmacological understandings may easily lead to inadequate pain treatment.

DIFFICULTIES MANAGING POST-OPERATIVE PAIN

When a surgical incision is made, it cuts through various tissues and nerve endings. Specific nociceptors are activated, as are free nerve endings. Inflammatory mediators (bradykinin, serotonin, and histamine) are released, causative of peripheral sensitization. The patient will now present with hyperalgesia, the magnification of noxious signals. These signals are broadcast to the dorsal horn of the spinal cord where they are amplified and increased in duration. Nociceptor signals and peripheral sensitization cause different fibers to transmit painful stimuli to the dorsal horn. Clinically, allodynia then occurs, a state of pain where non-painful (i.e., normally non-noxious) stimuli are perceived as painful. As signals enter the central nervous system from the periphery they will further increase in duration and intensity. Wind up or central sensitization now transpires. To successfully manage postoperative pain, both methods of pain signal transmission much be treated.

COMPLICATIONS OF UNMANAGED PAIN

Three **potential complications of unmanaged pain** are:

- **Atelectasis (lung collapse):** Can occur when pain is not managed appropriately. It is a frequent complication during the postoperative period. When the patient experiences pain while breathing, muscle splinting may occur. This may cause a decreased vital capacity, decreased functional residual capacity and finally decreased alveolar expansion and ventilation.
- **Postoperative pneumonia:** Often emerges when insufficient pain control makes coughing too difficult. Secretions may be retained, leading to postoperative pneumonia.
- **Cardiovascular compromise:** May be caused by the body's sympathetic response to pain. Tachycardia, increased peripheral resistance, and hypertension symptoms are linked to increased cardiac work and myocardial oxygen consumption. Myocardial infarction and ischemia are inherent dangers.

Five additional complications of **unmanaged pain** include:

- **Reduced mobility:** Arising from postoperative pain, increases the risk of deep vein thrombosis and pulmonary embolism. When patients remain immobile venostasis and platelet aggregation increase postoperative risks.
- **Decreased gastrointestinal motility:** Where both surgery and anesthesia combine with postoperative pain to decrease alimentary motility, particularly in the colon. This may lead to an ileus as a dangerous complication of postoperative pain.
- **Urinary retention:** Can also occur when postoperative pain is not managed well.
- **Electrolyte imbalance and hyperglycemia:** Where the endocrine system is affected by acute pain, sodium and water are retained and blood sugar levels may dangerously rise.
- **Psychological disturbances:** as there is always a psychological aspect to pain, postoperative pain may also cause psychological and emotional distress.

Pain Diagnoses and Syndromes

CRPS

Complex Regional Pain Syndrome (CRPS) was once known as Reflex Sympathetic Dystrophy Syndrome or RSDS, and may still be referred to as such by some clinicians. Two forms and three stages have been identified, although not all patients will progress through each stage.

- **CRPS Type I** typically develops after an injury or noxious event. There is no associated nerve injury. Pain is seemingly disproportionate to the initial event.
- **CRPS Type II** generally occurs in the hand or foot after a nerve has been injured. Injury to a nerve differentiates CRPS Type II from Type I.

Symptoms of CRPS are divided into stages:

- **Stage I symptoms** include burning pain, rapid nail and hair growth, muscle spasms, joint stiffness, and vasospasm.
- **Stage II symptoms** include worsening pain, edema, cyanosis, muscle atrophy, cracked and brittle nails, allodynia or hyperalgesia, and marked osteoporosis.
- **Stage III symptoms** are characterized by irreversible changes in muscles and skin. Severe pain continues, along with profound muscular atrophy, flexor tendon contractures, and severe osteoporosis.

Signs and Symptoms

Complex Regional Pain Syndrome is characterized by a continual burning pain in an extremity after what seems to be a minor trauma. Allodynia or dysesthesia are also present. Complex regional pain syndrome is related to sympathetic hyperactivity. Vasodilatation with amplified temperature of the affected limb, excessive sweating and edema may occur initially. Occasionally the skin of the appendages may atrophy and become cool, red and clammy. As complex regional pain syndrome progresses it may cause disuse which will cause atrophy of the bone (demineralization). As the syndrome progresses the patient may experience persistent coldness, pallor, cyanosis, Raynaud phenomenon, atrophy of the skin and nails, loss of hair on the affected area, tissue atrophy and joint stiffness. Complex regional pain syndrome is aggravated by use of the extremity and symptoms are relieved by immobilization. Patients may not present with all these symptoms at once and additional limbs may be affected.

Children

Complex regional pain syndrome is more common in females than males and it is more frequently found in the lower limbs. It is rarely seen in children under the age of nine. Symptoms are similar in children and adults. **Children** are able to identify a precipitating injury before the onset of symptoms and can sometimes develop similar symptoms in a second extremity with no precipitating injury. Complex regional pain syndrome is often found in children who place a lot of pressure on themselves. Often, they are involved in highly competitive sports and many patients also experience eating disorders. The severity of the pain symptoms can be amplified by anxiety and stress. It is important for parents and children affected by complex regional pain syndrome to understand that the pain symptoms being experienced are not caused by injury, rather the cause is a defect in pain signal transmission.

Fibromyalgia Syndrome

Fibromyalgia syndrome is defined as musculoskeletal pain and aching that is diffuse and associated with stiffness and expected tender points, where no underlying physiological condition is found. There is still debate as to whether FMS is a single entity or several pain syndromes with related characteristics. The American College of Rheumatology defines FMS with these criteria: widespread pain involving three bodily sites for three months or longer, and the elimination of any conditions that may cause comparable pain and presence. Also, reproducible tenderness at eleven out of eighteen established fibromyalgia sensitivity points.

Persons suffering from fibromyalgia syndrome suffer from widespread, continuous pain that can vary in severity from day to day, stiffness with outer range of motion (as well as stiffness in the morning), and possibly chronic exhaustion. Sleep disturbances, memory loss, migraine headache and irritable bowel are also clinical features of FMS.

Relationship of Pain to Suffering

The International Association for the Study of Pain defines pain as "an unpleasant **sensory and emotional experience** associated with actual or potential tissue damage, or described in terms of such damage." Thus, pain is considered a physiological and emotional reaction to the sensation a person is feeling. Pain will always include a **subjective element.** A person experiencing pain may experience both physical and psychological components. Both will need to be dealt with to treat the pain effectively. Suffering is a significant awareness of pain, injury or loss. Suffering is not considered a measure of pain or distress itself. Rather, suffering is how a person responds to the impression of pain. There is no calibrated measure of pain, because it is felt and described differently by every person.

Pain Descriptors and Characteristics

QUALITY PAIN ASSESSMENT

COMPONENTS

A **quality pain assessment** includes the following:

- **Location of the pain.** This may be the most important factor in diagnosing the underlying cause of a patient's pain. Using photographs, ask the patient to show where their pain is, or have them point to it on their own person. Have the patient also describe where their pain is felt. This may help reveal pain that is not localized, or pain that radiates, travels, or otherwise changes.
- **Describing the pain.** Have the patient use their own words to describe the pain sensations they are experiencing. If the patient is having difficulty coming up with words to accurately describe their pain, offer them a set of words to choose from.

PAIN DURATION AND ALLEVIATING/AGGRAVATING FACTORS

A quality pain assessment addresses **pain duration and alleviating/aggravating factors** as follows:

- Determine the duration of pain. Ask the patient "When did the pain start?", "How long has it lasted or did it last?", "When was it worse?", "When was it better?" These are all useful open-ended questions to start a patient talking about the duration of their pain.
- Identify alleviating and aggravating factors. Ask the patient "Are there things that make the pain worse?" (e.g., movement, coughing, pressure, etc.), "Is there anything that makes the pain better?" (e.g., hot or cold, pressure, massage, immobilization, etc.).
- Ask about temporal characteristics. "Is the pain worse in the morning or evening?", and "What treatments or medications have best reduced the pain?" Be sure to include questions about nontraditional methods of pain reduction (e.g., herbs, meditation, alcohol, etc.).

PAIN INTENSITY

A complete pain evaluation includes measures of **pain intensity**. There are many pain assessment tools designed to help the nurse and patient convey information accurately. Choosing a pain rating tool that best suits the patient's age, cognitive ability, culture and language is important. The nurse should then determine the range of pain a patient experiences by asking the patient to rate their current pain level, best and worst estimate of pain etc., using the selected tool. A realistic goal of tolerable pain intensity should also be set using the same pain assessment tool. Finally, the same tool should be used by all involved health care providers to provide continuity in care and to increase the likelihood of successful pain management.

PAIN ASSESSMENT

There are many barriers to the effective treatment of pain. An inadequate **pain assessment** is one of them. If a thorough pain assessment is not done the information needed to treat the pain will be absent, and treatment may then be unsuccessful. A pain rating scale should be used on admission, and the same scale should be used throughout the course of therapy and by all staff who care for the patient. Scale use consistency will help nursing staff to better identify a baseline and subsequent changes in intensity of pain. Information from subjective and observational pain assessments also should be utilized in formulating a treatment plan. During an observational assessment, care must be used to identify any cultural, gender, or personal barriers the patient may use to mask their pain. However, an observational assessment is meant to complement, not replace, a full pain assessment.

Pain History

ACCURATE AND PERTINENT MEDICAL HISTORY

A **pertinent medical history** is an important part of a nursing pain assessment. Information gained from a person's medical and surgical history is also invaluable in planning for pain management. Any past experiences with pain should be specifically explored, as well as past or current chemical use or abuse. A detailed medication history should be taken and all surgeries and medical disorders listed as well. Special attention should be given to any therapies, procedures, surgeries or medications that could be related to the pain the patient is experiencing now. Patients in pain do not always notice connections between past medical events and the situation they are in now. A thorough medical and surgical history can help connect those experiences.

PAIN ASSESSMENT INTERVIEW PROCESS

To obtain accurate information through a chronic pain assessment instrument, the nurse must have knowledge of the associated **interview process.** Subtleties in how an assessment tool is presented to the individual can have a significant impact on the information that is produced during the interview. Prior to the interview the nurse should review the chart and establish a comfortable environment in which the interview will take place. Finding a setting that is quiet, private and accessible is a difficult task in most hospitals. However, doing so will significantly improve and increase the quality of the information given. In opening the interview, establish oneself early on as willing to help, courteous and interested in the individual, their family and their needs.

VALUE OF INTERVIEWING SKILLS

The **interview component** of a pain patient assessment is an integral part of the history and physical examination. Only by way of the interview can certain essential data be gathered. Information gained during the interview process can help with the diagnostic impression and formulation and is also invaluable in helping to better define the patient's pain experience and his or her response to pain and illness, both of which are factors known to greatly impact the pain experience. Creating an atmosphere where communication can openly and easily occur is imperative to gaining adequate and useful information. Patients who are not engaged in a trusting, accepting way are less likely to be forthcoming with details that could greatly affect the success of treatment.

BEGINNING AND CONDUCTING THE PAIN ASSESSMENT INTERVIEW

When **beginning and conducting a pain assessment interview**, nurses should:

- Greet the patient in proper form (Mr., Ms., Mrs.) unless instructed to do otherwise, or speaking with an adolescent or child.
- Address the patient's immediate comfort before beginning the interview process (e.g., seating, lighting, tissues, etc.). Use open ended questions that will allow the patient to give more elaborate and complete answers. For example, "What would you like to tell me about your back pain?"
- Listen actively. Remember, these individuals are in grave pain and under severe stress. Be attentive, give them time to answer, and do not rush them in anyway.

EXPECTED GENERAL DEMEANOR OF THE NURSE

While being interviewed, patients observe behavior and take **nonverbal cues f**rom their interviewer. Even when under time constraints, never present as hurried to the patient and family. Patients may consider this evidence that they and their pain are not important and that the nurse is not interested in helping them. Always appear calm and unhurried, providing the patient with a welcoming environment to discuss their most personal issues. Tactics such as teasing, using condescending behaviors or attitudes, as well as stereotyping and sarcasm are unacceptable in the interview process. Overt judgment of the patient and what they say must also to be left outside the interview arena.

INTERVIEWING TECHNIQUES

- **Facilitation**: Interviews are facilitated by active engagement including an attentive posture, consistent eye contact, and positive acknowledging statements to encourage the patient to say more.
- **Reflection**: Reflection is the practice of rephrasing and repeating the patient's thoughts back as they shared them. This helps both participants ensure that the information shared was received, and it encourages the patient to fill in the statements with more information.
- **Clarification**: Ask the patient to make elaborate on words or statements that are vague or unclear. Be clear in the request, saying something like, "Can you tell me what you mean?"
- **Empathic responses**: Respond to the individual and their family members in a way that demonstrates understanding and recognition of their statements and feelings.
- **Confrontation**: When the nurse witnesses behavior or statements displaying anger, anxiety or depression, they should be dealt with promptly when they come up.
- **Interpretation**: Taking information provided by the patient and making an inference ("If I understood you correctly, it sounds like that is really difficult to deal with."). Interpretive statements offered during the interview will serve to show empathy and to augment a mutual understanding.

ADDRESSING SENSITIVE TOPICS

There are many **sensitive topics** that an interviewer must cover in order to gain the information needed to adequately prepare and implement a treatment plan. Inquiring about alcohol and drug use is sensitive but essential to a pain assessment interview. Asking a patient "How much alcohol do you drink?" is preferred to "Do you drink alcohol?" The nurse is more apt to get a realistic answer. Remember, however, that everyone has a different view on how much is "too much." The answer to "Do you drink alcohol?" could be "Not much." When in reality the patient consumes six to eight beers every evening. Thus, have the patient be specific about quantities used.

OBTAINING ACCURATE INFORMATION

Four useful **interview methods** to improve information accuracy include the following:

- Ask the patient to give information in a chronological manner. Asking "What happened then?" or "What did you do after that?" will encourage them to continue providing useful information.
- In addition to using open ended questions ("Can you tell me about your headaches?") an interviewer should also utilize direct questions to extract important details. For example, "Can you describe your pain for me?" or "Does the pain stay here in your back or go elsewhere?" These kinds of questions will elicit more pointed and specific answers.
- When using direct questions do not lead the patient with statements. For example, "Does your pain shoot down your right side when it comes?" as compared with, "Does your pain travel at all?"
- When directing the interview and asking questions, use plain words that are understandable to the patient and their family members.

SUBJECTIVELY AND OBJECTIVELY GAINING INFORMATION REGARDING PHYSICAL ABUSE

During the interview process certain subtle behaviors may serve as **"red flags"** warning the interviewer that an individual is suffering from physical violence. For example, if the patient is being dominated during the interview by someone accompanying them, or if the person refuses to leave the room, those may be signs that there is physical violence occurring in the home. Often the person perpetrating the violence will appear anxious or concerned that the interviewer is questioning their loved one. During a physical exam look for bruising, burning or other physical signs of violence. If a nurse suspects violence, direct questioning may not work. Instead, they should say something like, "I have a lot of women tell me they're being abused at home. Is something going on at home you'd like to tell me about?" This allows the patient to more comfortably express their concerns.

BARKER & WHITFIELD'S CAGE QUESTIONS

Barker and Whitfield developed an interview acronym called **"CAGE"** to help interviewers obtain information about an individual's alcohol and drug use. Because everyone has different opinions regarding alcohol and drug use and because it is generally regarded as a taboo topic the CAGE questions can be particularly helpful:

- C: "Have your family members or friends ever *criticized* your drinking?"
- A: "Has that criticism ever *annoyed* you?"
- G: "Have you ever felt *guilty* about your drinking?"
- E: "Have you ever had a drink in the morning as an *eye-opener*?"

SEXUAL HISTORY

Asking questions about a **patient's sexual history and sexual health** can be very uncomfortable for both parties. It is usually best to wait until late in the interview to discuss these questions, giving the patient time to develop trust before delving too deeply. Always begin by asking permission to interview the individual about their sexual health and history. If they would rather not discuss sexual topics at this time, do not proceed. Asking them again after additional interactions or after more time has elapsed may prove more fruitful. Never make assumptions regarding a person's sexual orientation, preferences, marital status or attitudes toward pregnancy and contraception. Let them directly state what they believe and about their own views and personal practices.

INTERVIEWS WITH CHILDREN OVER THE AGE OF FIVE

Children five years of age and older can be interviewed with or without their parents present. The interviewer is more likely to get accurate information from the child who is five years of age or older, as they are able to share much of their history and can usually describe their pain more accurately than their parents. Call the child by the name, use eye contact and attending and sympathetic facial expressions, and convey warmth. Using open ended questions and language that is familiar to the child will be most helpful. For example, "Your mommy says you get headaches. What can you tell me about them?" And, "Do your headaches worry you?" Also, "Can you show me exactly where it hurts?"

INTERVIEWS INVOLVING PARENTS OF PATIENTS

Interviewing a patient who is an infant or child will necessarily involve the **parents** and/or caregivers of the child. Closely observe the interactions between the parents and the child to better understand how they relate to each other. Be aware that some information sharing and questioning should not take place in the presence of the child, and plan and respond accordingly. Use the same principals of questioning (i.e., open ended questions to illicit information, and direct questions to quantify information and gain particular data) as used with adult patients. Revise only the vocabulary and interrogatory style used. Put questions to the child when possible, recognizing that parents may sometimes respond with their own biases, assumptions, perceptions and needs in mind. Always refer to an infant or child by name.

OBSTACLES WHEN INTERVIEWING PEDIATRIC PATIENTS

Assessing the **pediatric patient** for pain presents unique obstacles. Children experience pain the same as adults. However, their pain is often overlooked. For example, children who suffer from disease process with a known pain component may not be asked routinely about their pain. A good rule of thumb is: "if it is painful for an adult, it is painful for the child," and the pain inquiry process should be carried out similarly. Children who are young or who have developmental delays may have particular difficulty communicating their pain, often making the assessment process more difficult than the treatment. Interacting with adults is very different than interaction with children, and this puts the pediatric patient at great risk for untreated and under-treated pain.

DEVELOPMENTAL EXPECTATIONS RELATED TO PEDIATRIC PAIN ASSESSMENT

Developmental processes related to pain assessment include the following:

- Infants are completely dependent on caregivers and clinicians to accurately assess their pain. Because they are nonverbal their behavior must be observed closely. Infants in pain may exhibit pain behaviors such as: crying, grimacing, eye squeezing, chin quivering, and withdrawal of limbs, hypertonicity and touch aversion.
- Adult pain scoring tools are usually beyond a toddler and school-aged child's cognitive abilities. Toddlers can typically report only that pain is present or absent. Some very small children may be able to localize their pain.
- School aged children are cognitively able to describe their pain to an interviewer.
- By the time a child reaches adolescence they should have the ability to use adult pain assessment tools.
- Children experience significant stress during times of illness and pain and this may cause them to regress to an earlier developmental stage.

PAIN IN CHILDREN IN PREOPERATIONAL DEVELOPMENTAL STAGE

A **preoperational child** (ages two to seven years old) sees pain as a magical or mystical entity. They do not have the ability to recognize cause-and-effect, and will only interpret pain as an immediate physical experience. They do not understand the relationship of pain to pain relievers or analgesia. A preoperational child may also perceive pain as punishment for something they did or did not do. Because they do not understand the causes underlying their pain, they may hold someone responsible and react in a physically aggressive manner. Remind the preoperational child that they are not being punished with pain. Use language that a young child will understand. For instance, "boo-boo" and "owie" are appropriate word substitutions for pain, as young children may not understand the word *pain* as it relates to a particular sensation.

PAIN AND THE CONCRETE-OPERATIONAL CHILD AND THE TRANSITIONAL-FORMAL CHILD

Between the ages of **seven and twelve** children are becoming immersed in school and learning new things. Age-appropriate explanations about pain should take into consideration the fact that these children have a basic understanding of their body and its internal organs, and are fearful of bodily harm. Supporting them and reassuring them regarding their fears is important for successful pain assessment and treatment. Basic, understandable, and empathetic explanations regarding their medical situation and pain should be given until an understanding is achieved. Around ten to twelve years old children start to understand cause and effect. "When I do this, then that happens."

This understanding in the transitional-formal child is helpful because these children can see that even difficult treatments may result in less pain, thus they are more likely to cooperate.

Pain and the Formal-Operational Child

Children in the **formal-operational developmental stage** (those older than twelve years of age) have begun early problem solving. However, they do not have the maturity of an adult in problem solving; this will not emerge until well into adolescence. Thus, formal-operational children need additional support and information about their treatment plan (i.e., tell them what tests, procedures, medications and interventions are planned for their care). When under stress these children will need still further support. Decompensation and regression are common, resulting in an inability to use even the limited resources available to them for coping with their pain. Thus, while children can gradually begin to look and act like adults, they are not and need to be treated within their developmental parameters.

Obstacles During Pain Assessment Interview with Adolescents

As an interviewer, questioning a **teenager** will present specific obstacles. For example, establishing a rapport may be more difficult. Showing a teenager empathy and genuine interest will help maintain the interview process. Be sure to clarify the concept of confidentiality as it relates to what they share and what is told to them. There may be certain sensitive topics that will need to be discussed with both the patient and their parents. Clarify this in advance, and be sure to involve the teenager in that process. Asking occasional questions about the adolescent's hobbies, friends, sports or other activities will help keep the conversation focused on the teenager rather than the problems involved. Make every effort to keep the environment inviting and friendly.

Unique Obstacles with Adolescents

The following are **four roadblocks** to a successful adolescent pain assessment interview:

- The practice of **repeating the patient's statements** back to them in an attempt to draw out more information and establish understanding is often ineffective with adolescents who are cognitively immature. It may become a source of confusion rather than a way to clarify understanding.
- Using **silence** to try and elicit responses to questions is also often ineffective and inappropriate. Adolescents may interpret this as disengagement, disinterest or manipulation, rather than as time for further introspection.
- Many adolescents have a difficult time **discussing their feelings** with adults, and this may make the interview process particularly challenging. Establishing an inviting, comfortable, private, and safe environment will help put the teenager at ease and make conversing more natural.
- **Confronting adolescents** will only serve to cause anxiety and defensiveness. They are then also more likely to avoid the questions being asked, often derailing the interview completely.

Unique Obstacles with Aging Patients

Interviewing the **elderly or aging patient** presents some unique obstacles. Often, their vision and/or hearing can be impaired, causing difficulty in understanding and communication. Information processing delays also become more apparent as we age. Giving elderly individuals more time to answer will help them adequately process the questions and provide more accurate answers. Further, have the elderly or aging patient help establish goals and priorities for the interview. This can help them better anticipate the information needed and more fully prepare adequate responses. Elderly or aging patients have a long history, and learning how they responded in the past to crisis may help now. Finally, be sure to assess for activities of daily living and safety in their home, as well.

CLOSING A PAIN ASSESSMENT INTERVIEW

When **bringing an interview to a close,** ask an open-ended question to sum up the interview. For example, ask the individual if they have anything further to add that hadn't yet been discussed. Questions such as, "Do you have anything to add?" or "Is there anything we haven't gone over?" are both good choices. Clarifying for the patient what will happen next in their treatment plan is important. This emphasizes to them what will be done with the information gained in the interview, and who it will be shared with. Write down any instructions had for them, and include the names and numbers of other individuals they may need to contact, along with personal contact information.

Pain Assessment Techniques, Scales, and Tools

FIFTH VITAL SIGN

Pain is now considered the **fifth vital sign**. Joint Commission guidelines integrate pain measurements into charting at the bedside, in addition to mapping a patient's classic vital signs: temperature, blood pressure, heart rate and respiratory rate. When assessing pain, it is important not to simply rely on the visual analog scale or a verbal rating scale. Neither of these tools discriminates between pain at rest and pain with movement or incidental pain. These types of pain are more difficult to control. Following a patient's actual response to their analgesic management under varying conditions is also important. Side effects such as sedation, nausea and vomiting, respiratory depression and cognitive impairment are as important to note as pain control. Pain must be assessed and managed properly in the postoperative period to decrease unfavorable outcomes.

UNIDIMENSIONAL VS. MULTIDIMENSIONAL PAIN ASSESSMENT TOOLS

Unidimensional pain assessment tools measure a single element of pain (i.e., intensity). When the cause of pain is known, they are very helpful. Most unidimensional tools were developed for use in research and for accumulating statistics.

Multidimensional pain assessment tools are designed to address two or more dimensions of pain. They gauge not only intensity but also the nature and location of the pain as well. Because pain negatively impacts activity levels and mood, these tools may also evaluate these complications. While designed for self-report, they can be integrated into an interview process. Used more commonly with chronic pain, they can also be effectively used when acute pain becomes prolonged.

UNIDIMENSIONAL PAIN ASSESSMENT TOOLS
NUMERIC RATING SCALE

A **numeric rating scale** uses numbers to rate pain, with 0 being no pain, 5 being moderate pain, and 10 being the worst pain. The numerals are arranged along a line from 0 to 10. This test can be administered either visually or verbally. It has also been validated in chronic pain patients, trauma, cancer and illiterate patients. As with any assessment tool requiring a patient response, teaching is required. The patient should be educated about how often their pain should be assessed, and how to provide consistent comparative responses to the ordinal scale. The patient should also understand that they have a responsibility to communicate and to set and meet goals both for acceptable pain levels and expected activity levels as well.

The numeric rating scale is quick and simple to use, and culturally and linguistically unbiased. Critics feel that it oversimplifies the pain experience. Regardless, the measurement the patient gives to their pain is easy to compare with earlier ratings, the rating scale can be used with other languages, and it offers a consistent format for use throughout a facility. When used with patients who are not reliable or are nonverbal it has a decreased validity, and it is not user friendly for patients who suffer from higher levels of cognitive impairment. The scale is also less reliable when used with patients who have visual or auditory impairments.

Simple Verbal Descriptive Scale

A simple **verbal descriptive scale** is a continuum line with six distinct phrases used to describe pain. The phrases: "no pain" (none), "mild pain" (mild), "moderate pain" (discomforting), "severe pain" (distressing), "very severe" (horrible), "worst possible" (excruciating) are placed in equal increments along a line. The patient can verbally or visually report their pain intensity in relation to the key phrases used. This tool is both fast and easy to use as well as being easy to score and to compare with previous pain ratings. However, it is difficult for very old or very young patients to use, as well as being problematic for those who are cognitively impaired. Further, it is not easily translated to alternative languages as discrepancies in actual phrasing may occur in the translation process.

VAS

The **Visual Analogue Scale (VAS)** is a unidimensional pain rating system that asks patients to make marks on a line calibrated with pain descriptions. Options range from "No pain" to "Pain as bad as you have ever experienced." This approach allows the questioner to evaluate the efficiency of the patient's pain treatment. The descriptors may also be revised to "less severe", "unchanged" and "more severe" descriptions on the line. This can give the practitioner a comparative view in evaluating pain relief success. This approach is also relatively unbiased in nature. However, it is visually based and thus those with sight impairments could not use it independently. Translation would be required for non-English speakers, whereas numerical ratings can typically be used regardless of the language spoken. Finally, total illiteracy would also be a barrier.

Visual analogue scales are easy to use, quick, highly sensitive and easy to interpret. The results are simple to compare to previous readings. This scale is also easily translated to other languages and for others to score without reading the alternate language. Visual analogue scales are considered reliable tools for research as well as being among the best tools for assessing variations in pain intensity. It is, however, difficult for very young and old patients to comply with, as well as patients who are dealing with a cognitive dysfunction, post-surgical patients, or patients suffering from dementia. It has been validated for use with patients in chronic pain, those with rheumatic disease, and with children older than five years of age.

Wong-Baker Faces Pain Rating Scale

The **Wong-Baker faces pain rating scale** is a sequence of caricature faces ranging from smiling (no hurt) to a crying face (hurts worst). The patient is expected to point to the face that looks like what they are feeling. The Wong-Baker faces are considered by some to be easier than either a numeric rating tool or a visual analogue scale. These faces are often used with pediatric patients because there is no need for reading or verbal skills. This scale is generally acceptable for use with a child older than three years of age. Because the faces are depicted as cartoon characters, there is no culture, gender or ethnic bias associated with the tool, although sad or crying faces are not wholly accepted in every culture. Another problem with the faces is that there is sometimes confusion for the patient, determining whether to report their mood versus their pain experience.

Oucher Pain Rating Scale and Poker Chip Method

The **Oucher pain rating scale** and the **Poker Chip method** of pain assessment may be summarized as follows:

- The **Oucher pain rating scale** is a series of newborn faces (actual photographs vs. the cartoons seen in the Wong-Baker faces) that range from extreme distress to impartial. This tool can be used with most ages and can be made multicultural. It is easy to use and doesn't take much time. However, like the Wong-Baker faces it can sometimes cause misreporting of "mood" in lieu of "pain."
- With the **poker chip method of pain assessment,** a patient is given four poker chips, each symbolizing a "piece" of pain. The patient decides how many chips represent the amount of pain they are experiencing. This method is easy and quick. It does require a certain level of cognitive capacity, however, and would not be appropriate for those patients who are cognitively impaired or are nonverbal. It may be used with an interpreter.

Behavior Rating Scale

When patients are unable to report their own pain, a **behavior rating scale** is often used. Behavioral pain scales attempt to ascertain pain levels based upon observations of a patient's behaviors. Facial expressions, vocalizations (crying, moaning, whimpering, yelling out), movements and touch are all considered. There are a variety of behavioral scales used to accommodate differing developmental levels and situations. These scales are ideal tools for use with infants, nonverbal children, and cognitively impaired patients. However, as with any information obtained by a second-party in a subjective manner (i.e., with the provider judging and rating the behavior independently), this approach is inherently flawed. Behaviors can often poorly reflect a patient's pain, and other behaviors may be used to dismiss any evidence of pain. Thus, diligent and consistent efforts must be made to identify and treat pain in these challenging patients.

Body Diagram Method and Daily Diary Method

The **body diagram** and **daily diary pain assessment** tools may be summarized as follows:

- The **body diagram method** uses an outline of the body provided for the patient to identify locations of pain and then shade them in to indicate intensity. It is easy to use and can be used with an interpreter if there is a language barrier. However, the results are not easily compared with previous ratings and the tool is not suitable for the cognitively impaired.
- The **daily diary method** of pain assessment requires the patient to keep records regarding their pain over a period of time. This is easy for the patient to do, and it provides more in-depth information. Further, it often gives patients a feeling of control in the treatment of their pain. However, for the information to be useful, the patient must be motivated. Also, the tool would not be helpful for immediate treatment of pain, and it is not a tool to be used with those who are cognitively impaired.

Acute Pain Assessment Tools

Acute pain assessment tools may be used in emergency departments, urgent care settings, surgical units and other clinical areas. There is a need for them to be fast and easy to use and record in the medical chart. These tools need to be multicultural and multilingual and must provide options for those who are illiterate or young. The same acute pain assessment tool needs to be used in all departments and by all staff over the full course of a patient's inpatient treatment. Using a consistent tool to create an initial baseline and to reassess after treatment will provide the patient with the best chance of successful pain management. Have the patient discuss a realistic pain management goal, with the understanding that complete pain control may not be possible given their specific injury and treatment requirements.

> **Review Video: Assessing Pain**
> Visit mometrix.com/academy and enter code: 693250
>
> **Review Video: Assessment Tools for Pain**
> Visit mometrix.com/academy and enter code: 634001

ANGER ASSESSMENT

As may be expected, anger is broadly witnessed in individuals suffering from chronic pain. **Assessment of anger** through a multidimensional assessment tool and interview process should be mandatory for every chronic pain patient. Researchers Kerns and colleagues found that an individual's internalized feelings of anger strongly correlated to their pain intensity, the perceived burdensomeness of that pain, and the documented frequency of their pain behaviors. In highly debilitating cases, such as those where spinal cord injuries are present, pain is even more closely related to anger and hostility. The relationship between anger and pain exacerbation has not received enough research attention. However, one may expect that anger could be an exacerbating factor of pain as well as a hurdle in rehabilitation and disability management.

PSYCHOSOCIAL PAIN INVENTORY

One of the most frequently used tools designed specifically for interviewing pain patients is called the **Psychosocial Pain Inventory** or the PSPI. It consists of 25 open-ended questions asked of the individual and a family member about psychosocial aspects of the patient's pain experience. The primary topics covered are: major stressful life events, stressors related to pain, pain behaviors at home, prior painful or disabling medical problems, and family models of chronic pain coping. A standardized scoring system identifies factors that are most significant to the patient's pain. The test is administered by a psychologist and can take upwards of an hour and a half to two hours. This extended testing may significantly tire the patient, and cost may also be a factor in determining whether or not this testing is appropriate.

MULTIDIMENSIONAL PAIN ASSESSMENT TOOLS

INITIAL PAIN ASSESSMENT TOOL

The **Initial Pain Assessment Tool** is designed to be used at the time of patient admission as the first line of questioning regarding the patient's condition. Its comprehensive nature and adaptable format make it easy to use in different clinical areas, in keeping with continuity of care. The following components are included:

- Location of pain – body charts are included.
- Intensity of pain – different unidimensional methods may be used to assess intensity of pain, making the overall tool adaptable to different scenarios and populations.
- Quality of pain – elicits a description of pain.
- Onset, variations and rhythms – when pain is worse, better.
- Manner of pain expression – nurse's observation and patient's verbalization.
- What relieves the pain? – what has been done previously that has worked or not worked.
- What causes or increases the pain – identifying specific scenarios.
- Effects of the pain – physical, psychological, social and/or financial.
- Other comments – i.e., miscellaneous details.
- Plan – the resultant treatment plan.

MPQ

The **McGill Pain Questionnaire (MPQ)** is the most widely used tool for pain assessment. It has dual duties, being used as both a diagnostic aid and an instrument for pain management. It comes in both a short form (that measures sensory and affective dimensions of pain as well as pain intensity) and a long form (that measures pain location, pattern of pain over time, sensory and affective dimensions of pain, and pain intensity). It is administered both verbally and visually. The tool is used to collect information pertaining to diagnosis, medication use, pain and medical history, other symptoms and specific defining features. It also contains a list of words describing pain that are subdivided into three groups: sensory, affective, and evaluation. It is available in several languages.

Advantages and Disadvantages

There is a multitude of studies and research to support the validity of this tool. It is considered the gold standard. It is designed to detect changes in the pain experience as well as the sensory, affective, and evaluative dimensions of the patient's pain experience. In its short form only two to three minutes are needed to complete it.

The long form does take thirty minutes to complete and requires concentration. It will not be acceptable for use with someone who is significantly cognitively impaired. Some of the descriptive terms used can also be inaccurately used to imply intensity. The tool does not include measures for decreased function, nor complaints regarding pain. Nor does it address any somatic interventions that have been tried or may yet be desired. Finally, it does not evaluate the level of function that the individual has remaining.

BPI

The **Brief Pain Inventory (BPI)** was developed to assess pain in cancer patients, and is now used in other diseases as well. The BPI focuses on gathering information about pain and its impact on daily functioning. Information collected includes: severity of pain, impact of pain on daily activities, pain location, pain medications, and the patient's report of pain relief in the last week or 24 hours. Requiring only about ten minutes to complete (the short version takes only five minutes), it is available in many languages. Because it was developed initially for cancer patients, the interviewer should be aware of questions that don't exactly reflect what the individual is experiencing.

Advantages and Disadvantages

The most significant advantage of the Brief Pain Inventory (BPI) is that it effectively addresses the multidimensionality of pain. It assesses the patient's location, intensity and blueprint of pain, while also reporting on medications, pain relief, patient beliefs, and the effect the patient's pain has had on their quality of life. It can be reliably translated into other languages without losing the integrity of the tool. However, it does require cognitive skills to complete and is not appropriate for the use with the very young or someone who is cognitively impaired. Another flaw lies in some response options delimited by restrictive top and bottom parameters, leading to reduced patient representation in the tool.

MPI

Originally, the **Multidimensional Pain Inventory (MPI)** was the West Haven-Yale Multidimensional Pain Inventory (WHYMPI). A 64-item tool, it is designed for individuals to self-report their pain experience. There are three parts and twelve subscales. The first two parts include the patient's consideration of their pain process, pain's impact on their daily lives, the patient's perception of their support systems, and several other aspects. Part three focuses on determining how frequently the individual performs 18 common daily activities. Three distinct profiles are derived from this information: dysfunctional, interpersonally distressed, and adaptive coper. This tool can be translated into several languages without difficulty.

MMPI AND THE STATE-TRAIT ANXIETY INVENTORY

The **MMPI** and **State-Trait Anxiety Inventory** can be summarized as follows:

- The **Minnesota Multiphasic Personality Inventory (MMPI)** can help identify the psychological attributes of an individual's pain experience. Hypochondriasis, depression and hysteria can all contribute to pain perceptions and experiences, and this tool aids in identifying individuals with those personality traits. This information can then be used to better help alleviate their perceived pain.
- The **State-Trait Anxiety Inventory** recognizes pain as a symptom in fear syndromes. Pain can be the cause of anxiety, and anxiety can inflate somatic complaints particularly when the cause of the pain is unclear. Understanding that high levels of anxiety can serve to increase pain, and identifying those individuals who are prone to anxiety, can better help a nurse treat these individuals. This tool allows for the measurement of anxiety as it relates to pain, thereby helping to facilitate treatment plan formulation.

DARTMOUTH QUESTIONNAIRE

The **Dartmouth Pain Questionnaire** incorporates parts of the McGill Pain Questionnaire into an easily administered five-part tool. Those parts are: pain location (with a diagram), pain description (using words taken from McGill Pain Questionnaire), self-perception of pain, pain recording (this section can be used as a daily diary) and daily activities. This test does require patient instruction before it is administered and it is fairly complex in its scoring. However, it does elicit excellent information on an individual's remaining function, difficulties the patient is experiencing due to pain, and it produces a useful ratio of these functions and difficulties. This information can be meaningfully used to help explore and improve a chronic pain sufferer's functioning in their daily life.

UAB PAIN BEHAVIOR SCALE

Within the **UAB Pain Behavior Scale**, pain-related behaviors are scored for frequency: none, occasional and frequent. The following behaviors are evaluated: verbal statements, nonverbal cues, time spent lying down each day due to pain, facial grimaces, standing posture, mobility, body language (grasping or rubbing site of pain), use of assistive devices such as braces, crutches, cane, or using furniture to assist in mobility (these are not scored if prescribed as part of the treatment plan), TENS unit use, stationary movement (does the patient sit or stand still, or occasionally shift position?) and analgesic medication use.

ADVANTAGES AND DISADVANTAGES

The UAB Pain Behavior Scale is versatile and offers many **advantages**. First, there is minimal training time needed to be able to accurately administer the test, although the reliability does increase as the interviewer becomes more familiar with the instrument. Second, this tool does not rely on self-report (objective information) and the results are clinically relevant to the treatment plan.

However, the UAB Pain Behavior Scale has certain **disadvantages** as well. They include: 1) the need for staff to regularly watch for pain behaviors (staff is not always present when pain is experienced), 2) the pain is not quantified directly in the results, and 3) it does not allow for associated behavior changes that are not related to pain or pain management. Perhaps the most significant disadvantage among these is the tool's reliance on staff observation, which does not allow for reliable continuity in measurement when the patient is discharged from inpatient care.

INFORMATION GAINED INDIRECTLY FROM PHYSICAL PAIN ASSESSMENTS

From the first interaction of patient and caregiver, the **physical assessment** should begin. Upon meeting, the patient's general health, weight, muscle bulk and grooming should be ascertainable. Their gait, as well as their attitude and behavior toward the exam and interview process should also be considered. Physical inspection of their skin, hair, nails, symmetry and range of motion should all be noted. Observing how the individual reacts to motion and movement is important information. Swelling, redness and the shape of the joints should be recorded. Affect and emotional responses to the exam are also meaningful. All of the information gained directly and indirectly through a physical pain assessment must be integrated into the bigger picture of how an individual is coping with their pain. It must also clarify their ability to function with activities of daily living and their associated symptoms.

PHYSICAL EXAM FOCUSED ON PAIN

Physically assessing an individual for pain will focus on the location of the pain, the direction and location of any referred pain, and the nature of the pain. Rebound pain should be assessed for by palpation as well as within an interview. Pain stimulated when assuming a weight bearing position should also be assessed. The pain interview may gradually lead to a particular set of disease processes or conditions. Specific assessments for suspected illnesses should also be included in the physical exam. The physical assessment of pain should be ongoing with inpatients (i.e., evaluating pain changes, ongoing treatments, and those medications the pain responds to best). Thus, assessment is not over after admission. Rather, a constant, accurate, pain-focused physical assessment should continue.

SPECIAL CONSIDERATIONS WHEN ASSESSING PEDIATRIC PATIENTS FOR PAIN

Including the parent in the **child's assessment** is essential. The child's history, prior medical experiences, and typical responses to pain is information only they can provide. The parent knows the child best; leave judgments and opinions at the door. Use a multidisciplinary approach to help the family and child better reach their pain control goals. Children may display specific behavioral changes when experiencing intense acute pain: lying on their side with legs flexed, not wanting to be moved or to move themselves, or rocking their head from side to side. Chronic pain may induce behavioral changes, such as irritability, depression, apathy, and flat affect.

ADEQUATELY ASSESSING PAIN IN ELDERLY PATIENTS

Assessment of the **elderly pain sufferer** should always include physical, functional and psychological factors. Complete a thorough history and physical examination, establish an accurate medical diagnosis, and procure a baseline description of the pain the patient is experiencing. During the physical exam, specifically assess the following: trigger points, inflammation, and neurological function (including autonomic systems, sensory and motor deficits, and any vague suggestion of neuropathic conditions or nerve injuries). Evaluate any history of trauma, as well as any sudden changes in the character of their pain. In elderly patients, these changes can signify deterioration of an existing condition, or a possible new injury. Elderly patients may experience gaps or failures in their memory, and depression, fatigue, or sensory impairments that may complicate the assessment and information gleaning process. They may also underreport pain because it is considered an expected and necessary part of the aging and/or disease process. Thus, remember to include family members or other caregivers as important collateral sources of additional information.

COMPLETE ASSESSMENT OF ELDERLY CHRONIC PAIN PATIENT

Many components must be included in assessing the **elderly chronic pain patient.** For example, evaluating an elderly person's function in daily life as it relates to their mobility and independence is important. Psychological evaluation is also imperative, as depression and pain are strongly linked. Cognitive impairment should also be considered in the elderly patient, with the value of the information provided by the patient judged within the context of their cognitive functioning. Use both qualitative and quantitative pain assessment scales when assessing the elderly chronic pain patient. Be sure to evaluate the chronic pain patient for signs and symptoms of delirium and dementia and be aware of the impact of such factors on information gained in the history and physical exam.

PAIN BEHAVIORS EMPLOYED BY NONVERBAL, ELDERLY CHRONIC PAIN PATIENT

Pain behaviors of **nonverbal elderly chronic pain patients** may include:

- **Noisy breathing** – This term describes patients who are breathing with a great deal of strain and effort. These respirations sound loud, harsh or gasping and they may include periods of rapid breathing or hyperventilation. Their breathing is a negative sounding noise generated during inspiration or expiration.
- **Negative vocalization** – This term describes a patient who is using noise or speech with a negative or disapproving tone, muttering, or other vocalized noises with a definitive unpleasant sound. The pace of the noise may follow a faster rhythm than the conversation, or it may manifest as a drawn-out moan or groan. These patients may also repeat words in expressions of hurt or pain with mournful tones.
- **Tense body language** – These patients may present with tension throughout their extremities, evidenced by rigid muscle tone, inflexibility and stiff movements. They may also wring their hands together or clench their fists. Their knees may be pulled up tightly toward their bodies. Their entire posture may look strained and inflexible.
- **Fidgeting** – Fidgeting refers to acts of restless, impatient motion. The patient may behave in a squirming or jittery fashion. Sometimes they may be trying to get away from pain or a painful stimulus in a certain area (i.e., sitting uncomfortably on knotted clothes, or something else underneath them, etc.). They may also tug, rub or forcefully touch a body part, indicating discomfort.
- **Sad facial expression** – This patient may exhibit a troubled look, or they may appear hurt, worried, lost or lonesome. Their appearance is distressed and their eyes are sunken. They may be crying or be tearful as well.
- **Frightened facial expression** – This term describes a patient who looks scared or concerned. They may also appear bothered, afraid or troubled in some way. Their expression may appear alarmed, with open eyes and a pleading face.
- **Frown** – This term describes an emotionally strained face. Scowling or stern looks are common additions. Their overall expression is displeased, while employing a frown, furrowed brow and/or down turned corners of the mouth.

FACTORS TO ASSESS IN ADDITION TO PAIN SYMPTOMS AND BEHAVIORS IN ELDERLY PATIENTS

There are many influences on an **elderly patient's willingness and ability to report pain**. Patients who experience pain are less likely to be involved in activities, have more frequent mood disturbances, demonstrate greater feelings of anxiety, and have a decreased appetite. Therefore, these other factors should also be considered when conducting a pain assessment. Documentation of a patient's mood, activity, and their caloric intake and sleep patterns should be maintained in a continuum-based (i.e., trend-tracking) fashion, along with notes regarding changes in function. Combining this information with self-reported pain and observed pain behaviors will give a more complete picture of an elderly patient's pain.

BEHAVIORS OF NONVERBAL, ELDERLY CHRONIC PAIN PATIENTS

Behaviors in the nonverbal, elderly chronic pain patient, indicating they are **not presently experiencing pain**, may include:

- **Content facial expression** – When not in pain, this patient may display a pleasant or calm looking face. They appear to be at ease, peaceful and/or serene. Their jaw is unclenched or even slack and they have a relaxed facial expression. Their bodies and faces carry a message of serenity and peace.
- **Relaxed body language** – This patient's hands may be found in an open, unclenched position. They may be cuddled up or stretched out in a restful position. Their muscles are not carrying extra tension and their joints are not carrying additional stress. They may look idle, laid back, and easy going.

PAIN ASSESSMENT OF CHRONIC PAIN PATIENTS WITH SHORT-TERM MEMORY IMPAIRMENT

Traditionally, a patient is asked to compare levels of pain at different points during the day, from day to day, and/or from event to event. However, patient suffering from **short-term memory impairment** will be unable to provide these comparisons accurately. In this situation, the current status or pain report is the most important in determining actual levels of pain and discomfort. Caregivers should be monitoring, questioning and observing pain behaviors every few hours so that an accurate picture of the patient's pain can be ascertained, followed, and successfully treated. Thus, health care providers should establish pain diaries or flow sheets to document, share and track this patient's pain and treatments.

Quality of Life and Functional Ability

QUALITY OF LIFE

USE OF CHRONIC PAIN ASSESSMENT TOOLS IN ASCERTAINING QUALITY OF LIFE

Quality of life is impacted by chronic pain on many levels. Thus, a complete assessment may be complicated and difficult to achieve. Some of the more obvious quality of life deficiencies may emerge when completing a pain interview and taking a basic medical history. These may include sleep dysfunction, compromised employment, and immobility. However, other more complex factors may need investigation with an in-depth evaluative instrument to be brought to light. Thus, chronic pain assessment tools like the Dartmouth Questionnaire, MPI, or McGill Questionnaire can be invaluable in identifying issues such as anxiety, depression, reduced function in daily life, and compromised social interactions, intimacy and personal relationship issues, etc.

IMPACT OF CHRONIC PAIN ON QUALITY OF LIFE

Chronic pain differs from acute pain in that it is not a self-limiting event. It is considered an enduring circumstance of life with no end in sight and serving no purpose. Patients suffering from chronic pain may have difficulty with personal relationships, including partners, spouses, children, family, and friends. Sleep disturbances, weight gain, loss of appetite and loss of libido plague chronic pain sufferers, further impacting their quality of life. Employment issues and job losses may become factors in coping with chronic pain. Anxieties about finances, insurance, and financial security typically ensue. Relaxation and leisure activities may suffer, as well, due to cost constraints, relationship pressures, and physical limitations. The dimensions of these problems can become catastrophic, with the potential for profound emotional, psychological and behavior difficulties. Assessment, treatment and long-term management of pain should encompass all of these factors.

FOUR DOMAINS OF WELL-BEING

The **four domains of well-being and pain management** may be summarized as follows:

1. **Physical well-being.** Here we are considering not only the physical perception of pain, but also side effects of pain management treatments and the debilitating effect of pain itself. Nausea, anorexia, and fatigue are all associated with chronic pain and decrease quality of life.
2. **Psychological well-being.** Addressing how the pain patient is coping psychologically is important in assessing their overall quality of life. Anxiety, depression and any decrease in coping skills must be evaluated.
3. **Social well-being.** Pain can have a profound effect on one's personal relationships, particularly affecting sharing, sexuality and intimacy.
4. **Spiritual well-being.** Patients dealing with pain may also struggle with feelings of hopelessness and a great amount of suffering.

ADDITIONAL ELEMENTS IMPORTANT IN ASSESSING FOR QUALITY OF LIFE

Four **additional elements important in assessing for quality of life** are:

- **Physical functioning** – as it relates to mobility (or immobility) and independence is significant in determining an individual's quality of life. Without physical functioning, many other quality-of-life domains are compromised.
- **Cognitive function** – decisional capacity, mental alertness, comprehension, and attention are important elements for determining the self-efficacy, safety and related quality of life of an individual.
- **Individual perception** – the elements of a quality life are personal and unique to each individual; thus, quality of life must be assessed individually and specifically, rather than being assumed.
- **Medical and diagnostic situation** – the quality of life of a chronically ill or a dying patient needs to be assessed within the physical and emotional parameters of their medical situation. Comfort and pain control, as well as successful coping, are imperative to every patient's quality of life.

FUNCTIONAL CAPACITY ASSESSMENT

An evaluation tool developed by **Ware** uses a **36-item format short-form health survey** to measure health outcomes from the viewpoint of the patient. Within the 36 items, the patient will answer questions pertaining to their perception of physical function, their role physically, bodily pain and their general health. Vitality, social functioning and their emotional role are each evaluated, as well as their own report on their mental health and the health transition they've made. Viewing functional capacity through the perception of the patient is valuable in ascertaining the individual's true functional ability. Knowing where an individual needs assistance can be vital in helping them achieve greater independent and assisted function in their daily lives.

ASSESSMENT OF EXTENDED IMPACT OF PAIN ON LIFE AND MOOD

The **extended impact on an individual's life** also needs to be assessed as an integral part of the pain evaluation process. If an individual becomes unable to perform activities of daily living, is compromised at work, or becomes socially limited, the impact on their quality of life can be significant. Reciprocally, the pain the individual experiences may also be aggravated by losses of leisure activity, productivity, mobility and intimacy in personal relationships. An individual's mood may also be directly related to their ability to function in their daily life, including supporting themselves financially, and enjoying recreational activities and physical and emotional intimacy with their loved ones. Depression (along with anxiety) is strongly linked with chronic pain and therefore should always be evaluated during a chronic pain assessment.

Relationship Between Depression, Anxiety, and Pain

Nearly 40% to 50% of patients suffering from chronic pain also suffer from **depression**. Research has failed to provide a profile for a so-called *pain-prone* individual. Extensive research has repeatedly found that pain precedes the development of depression, rather than following an already developed depressive state. Depression and chronic pain may also be related in pathophysiology, as both experiences may involve the endogenous opiate systems of the body. Using multidimensional pain assessment tools will help unearth underlying anxiety and depression in the chronic pain patient. In addition, psychosocial services should be utilized to evaluate any potential need for therapy. Some pain anti-depressants have been successful in concurrently treating chronic pain and depression.

Depression Inventory Tools

While there is a known significant relationship between pain and depression, there is little agreement on the degree of depression as related to different pain states. Because depression may be masked by pain, and can be a response to pain as well, it is important to assess it thoroughly. Even so, there remains considerable diversity of opinion about the role of depression or depressed mood in the differential diagnosis of a chronic pain syndrome. Regardless, using **depressive inventory tools** to assess depression in the chronic pain patient will help provide the information needed to determine whether or not these patients are in a grave emotional state, and if further evaluation and treatment is essential. Identifying depression in the chronic pain patient is important to improving their quality of life, as well as the success of their treatment.

Stress Assessment

Using a multidimensional pain assessment tool appropriately will typically reveal other problems associated with chronic pain. **Stress** can both be a precipitating agent of chronic pain as well as a byproduct of such pain. Individuals suffering from stress-exacerbated chronic pain will need to learn coping strategies that help them successfully deal with life's stressors. Learning to recognize stressful situations and individual responses to those situations will help patients suffering from chronic pain reduce their physical responses to stress, decreasing the additional damage stress can cause. Referral for psychiatric evaluation and counseling may also be appropriate. Individuals who are struggling with chronic pain and stress should also be re-evaluated after appropriate interventions have been initiated so that continual treatment adjustments can be made.

Assessment and Management of Sleep Disturbances

Using a multidimensional pain assessment tool accurately will often bring to light certain other problems the individual is experiencing related to their pain that may be treatable. For example, **sleep disturbances** are common side effects of chronic pain. In addition, poor sleep can add to overall body pain. Therefore, in addition to a pain assessment, an overall psychosocial assessment should also be completed to reveal any sleep and/or other disturbances that may erode quality of life and ultimately impact the patient's pain. Input and interventions from different disciplines will often enhance treatment plans for both chronic pain and its side effects. Medications may be an appropriate treatment for some pain and poor sleep sufferers, while they and others may benefit greatly by learning specific relaxation techniques.

Assessment of Anorexia, Immobility, and Fatigue

Chronic pain is a multifaceted condition that when untreated can cause multiple major complications, many of which can weaken individuals and hasten death. **Anorexia, immobility and fatigue** are included among those complications. Anorexia, immobility and fatigue should be assessed with a multidimensional pain assessment tool and through an interview process for all patients presenting with chronic pain. Opioid management of pain should take place, as well as treatments for any anorexia, immobility and fatigue. Multiple versatile modalities should be incorporated into the treatment plan, where needed, to increase success. All identified associated symptoms should be continuously reevaluated as part of ongoing chronic pain treatment.

Assessment of Sexual Dysfunction

Assessing for all concurrent problems in a person with chronic pain is essential for their quality of life. Using a multidimensional pain assessment tool and an in-depth interview process will help bring light to each individual's struggles. Emotional, psychological and behavioral difficulties are often evident in individuals with chronic pain, making it likely that they are also experiencing **sexual dysfunction** or an interruption of their personal relationships and intimacy. Sexual function should be addressed near the end of an interview so that the patient first has adequate time to develop a trusting relationship with the interviewer. Always ask before proceeding with questions regarding sexual health and never make assumptions about marital status, sexual orientation, or sexual beliefs. Finally, never continue asking questions if the patient has refused permission to discuss the topic.

Assessing for Mobility Assistive Devices

Knowing how different **mobility assistive devices** work to increase balance can help determine which device would be best for any given individual. Canes, walkers and crutches can increase balance and make mobility more realistic. A walker is the most supportive of the devices. A walker without wheels (or with wheels on only two of the four legs) can be entirely self-supporting, allowing the patient to lean on the device to rest if needed. Walkers with wheels still offer some steadying support, but are easier to push along. A cane (whether single-point, four-point, etc.) can help an individual regain mobility and some independence, as it leaves one hand free for other tasks. Crutches are unstable and difficult to use, but they are ideal for an acute injury in an otherwise strong and healthy individual. Wheelchairs are most useful when they can be powered by the patient themselves. They are especially helpful in patients with bilateral lower limb weakness, lower body trauma or respiratory difficulty with exertion.

Associated Pain Components and Subjective Pain Experience

Associated pain components and **subjective pain experiences** should be addressed as follows:

- Determine any associated components of their pain. Nausea, vomiting and constipation are often more likely associated with pain and pain treatment than confusion, sedation, depression or anxiety. Ask the patients directly if they are suffering from any of these ailments.
- Determine a patient's subjective pain experience by asking about the impact of pain on the patient's life. How has the pain affected their sleep and rest cycles? Has their appetite increased or fallen off?
- Determine how their socialization and close relationships been affected by pain. Are they still able to interact with important others on a regular basis? How about sexual activity and intimacy? Is the patient able to complete their activities of daily living? Are employment and important hobbies already at risk?

All these areas are vital to maintaining a meaningful quality of life.

CULTURAL CONSIDERATIONS IN PAIN ASSESSMENT

Cultural considerations in pain assessment include the following:

- **Language barriers** – are destructive to quality care and treatment, and need to be overcome. Patients will not always acknowledge any lack of understanding (out of embarrassment, in an effort to be cooperative, or to avoid burdening caregivers). Thus, it is important not to assume language comprehension. Use interpreters as needed, and with careful regard to both gender and age (e.g., sexual problems may require a same gender interpreter, and an elderly patient may not be comfortable with a youthful interpreter).
- In certain cultures, **eye and/or physical contact** is disrespectful and inappropriate.
- **Personal space boundaries** are different in some cultures. Be respectful of any need to have only family members in the patient's personal space.
- **Cadence and rhythm of speech** differs from culture to culture. Silence may be regarded as a communicative understanding, or as respect.
- **Nonverbal cues** are important with language and cultural differences. Using nonverbal cues such as gestures and expressions will help in the assessment process.
- Many cultures are symbiotic with **spiritual and religious practices**. Allow time for rituals and prayers as needed.
- There are likely to be differences between provider and patient views.
- **Familial relationships** may be defined differently in many cultures. Specific roles such as caretaker, decision-maker or observer may also be culturally determined. Accept these roles as they are defined by the patient's culture, not one's own.
- Leave **judgments and opinions** regarding differing cultures outside of health care. Educate oneself on the impact that the patient's culture may have on their treatment plan, and organize accordingly. If their beliefs interfere with adequate pain resolution or treatment, offer consultation within the confines of patient privacy and then appropriate solicit other caretakers to help make decisions.

UNDERSTANDING CULTURAL DIFFERENCES AND BRIDGING GAPS WITH LANGUAGE BARRIERS

Patients who belong to a culture significantly different from that of their health care provider are faced with many challenges. Communication can be difficult, not only because of **language barriers** but also because of differing cultural norms. For example, certain cultural restrictions may govern the verbal or nonverbal expression of pain. In some cultures, pain can be associated with wrong doing and reacting to it may also be considered a weakness of character. Thus, shame may make it very difficult for some patients to admit their pain. Other cultures are prohibitively concerned about addiction as related to medicinal pain control. Those patients may not be willing to ask for analgesia to relieve their pain. In these situations, quietly initiating patient-controlled analgesia may be particularly helpful, allowing the patient to privately control their pain.

Coping Mechanisms and Support Systems

COPING

Generally, **coping** is the process of struggling to deal with difficulties, problems or responsibilities. Coping with pain refers to how a person deals with pain, adjusts to pain and reduces, minimizes the pain and stress related to pain. Coping behaviors may be unplanned. However, coping may also include purposeful and deliberate actions (including both overt and covert methods of coping).

- **Overt coping strategies** include rest, medication and the use of relaxation techniques to control pain.
- **Covert coping strategies** include methods of distraction, self-reassurance, problem solving, and trying to gain information to better cope with pain.

Using successful coping strategies can modify the way a person perceives pain as well as enhancing their ability to function well in everyday life.

IMPORTANCE OF MEASURING COPING SKILLS

Coping is defined as a continuous process that filters and responds to internal and external demands through cognitive and behavioral changes and efforts. In measuring pain coping skills, it is important to determine the ways that patients attempt to cope with their pain, and to evaluate the success of the coping skills they utilize. Also, it's important to ascertain what a patient believes about their pain and how those beliefs may be influencing their reactions. A patient's coping mechanisms are both conscious and unconscious, and some can be effective while others are not. What people believe about their pain (whether superstitious, religious, cultural, or philosophical) ultimately shapes their perception of pain and the outcome of their treatment.

COPING IN RELATION TO DEPRESSION AND ADAPTIVE FUNCTIONING

Coping in the wake of pain can be either advantageous or unfavorable, depending on the coping mechanisms used and how they are employed. When a patient utilizes active and **positive coping strategies**, such as distraction, engaging in engrossing activities, and ignoring pain sensations, adaptive functioning is more likely to occur. Depending on others for help or restricting one's activities (i.e., passive coping strategies) are approaches typically related to greater pain and depression. Educating patients on the likely outcomes of various coping strategies and their relationships to depression and pain intensity can ultimately enhance their capacity to cope well and better tolerate unexpected pain changes.

SURVEY OF PAIN ATTITUDES

Assessing the attitudes of chronic pain patients regarding their pain can greatly facilitate patient education and increase the use of advantageous coping strategies versus maladaptive ones. When patients are taught about productive coping, they are more likely to experience a decrease in the intensity of their pain and an increase in pain tolerance and overall well-being.

The **Survey of Pain Attitudes (SOPA)** is a tool that evaluates fifty-seven pain-related items, with each rated on a 5-point scale. Attitudes concerning control, disability, medical interventions, solicitude (expecting other to cater to their pain needs), medication, emotion and harm (defined as exercise avoidance) are all assessed. The SOPA instrument is widely used to measure beliefs and attitudes about pain and has been thoroughly researched. There have been multiple revisions to this tool and there are several versions (including two shorter versions) for clinical use.

CSQ

The **Coping Strategies Questionnaire (CSQ)** is a fifty-item instrument, and is the most widely used measure of pain coping strategies. Each item is scored on a 7-point scale in regards to frequency of use, and it evaluates seven specific coping strategies: six cognitive and one behavioral. Diverting attention from the pain, reinterpreting pain, self-statements regarding coping, ignoring the pain, using hope and prayer, catastrophizing and increasing activity despite pain are all measured with the CSQ. The Coping Strategies Questionnaire has been extensively used in research dealing with coping and adjustment. Other coping factors such as active and passive coping and flexibility of coping are additional measures to be considered.

VPMI

The **Vanderbilt Pain Management Inventory (VPMI)** is a self-report questionnaire containing nineteen items. The focus of the tool is to assess the frequency that chronic pain sufferers employ active or passive coping strategies when their pain intensity reaches moderate or severe levels. The tool evaluates cognitive coping and suppression, attention diversion, praying, and helpless mechanisms that the patient may use. This tool can successfully assess many of the coping mechanisms used by chronic pain sufferers and will aid in identifying active and passive dimensions of pain coping skills. It is not, however, prepared to assess those patients who are suffering from acute pain, intense pain, and pain with unpredictable dimensions.

IMPORTANCE OF COPING STRATEGY ASSESSMENT TO TREATMENT PLAN

Coping can be a conscious or unconscious process, as well as having maladaptive or favorable results. People dealing with chronic pain will find ways to deal with that pain, and assessing the coping techniques they are using may help to assist them in employing more effective techniques, as needed. If a patient is using maladaptive coping strategies, they are more likely to report greater levels of pain and decreased tolerance of that pain as well. Patients who are utilizing more effective coping strategies will report decreased pain intensity and increased tolerance to the pain. Thus, coping techniques are an important tool in helping the patient to manage their pain.

READINESS FOR CHANGE

Some chronic paint patients will see improvement over time while others never seem to have a change in their status. **Readiness for change** is likely a significant factor in this process. Knowing where the patient falls in the change process will help in planning appropriate interventions to promote behavioral change, encourage active participation in care, and increase chronic pain self-management skills. A powerful change agent helping patients understand that they can choose to change. Start with the question, "What do you want to change?" and follow this with, "What are you willing to do to get there?". Understanding that change takes sacrifice and work will help the patient to better understand and adhere to the change process.

INFLUENCE ON TREATMENT

The patient suffering from chronic pain is challenged by many obstacles. One of which is the way their behavior ultimately influences their eventual level of disability. Changing those behaviors that are incongruent with optimum functioning is difficult and a level of readiness must be assessed. Many factors may influence the patient's reluctance to change maladaptive behaviors. These include: unconscious conflicts, primary and/or secondary gains, personality disorders, psychopathology, insufficient education and/or poor alternate coping skills. To better understand and promote change in chronic pain behaviors, it may be helpful to utilize the Transtheoretical Model of change (TTM). It maps a series of stages that must be accomplished for a change in behavior to occur. How the patient responds to these stages will determine how ready they are to make behavioral changes, which in turn will impact their ultimate ability or disability.

TRANSTHEORETICAL MODEL OF CHANGE

The **transtheoretical model of change (TTM)** demonstrates how an accurate assessment of readiness to change is important. Certain interventions will not prove fruitful if presented to the patient before they are ready. For example, suggesting relaxation techniques to a patient in the precontemplation stage will backfire, as they are currently unwilling to make any changes in their behavior. At this stage, time would be better spent challenging their resistance to change by offering reasonable explanations and discussion. Thus, working within the patient's current stage will decrease frustration for both the patient and provider, and true progress is more likely to be achieved. Determining readiness to change may also reduce dropout rates and relapse occurrences in patients participating in chronic pain management programs.

The **first stage** in the TTM model is **"precontemplation."** Patients in this stage are extremely resistant to change and are not interested in making any adjustments or accommodations in their personal behavior for any reason, even to enhance treatment. These patients are often convinced that only external medical intervention will help them and that they can have no personal impact on their pain. They challenge any notion that their own behavior may be impacting their pain and are often described as: helpless, passive, and in extreme distress. These patients do not believe there is any psychological component to their pain.

The **second stage** in the TTM model is the **"contemplation"** stage. During this stage there is an increased awareness of personal responsibility for controlling pain. These patients are willing to at least consider the prospect that their own stress is impacting their pain process, and there may be things they can do behaviorally to better manage their pain. However, these patients are not yet committed to any change in their behavior. They are unsure if they can change, and they are equally unsure of how to create the needed changes. They are simply cultivating the idea of change and entertaining notions on how they might move forward. Even so, they are acknowledging that they are "stuck" and that something needs to change.

The **third stage** in the TTM model is **"preparation."** Patients suffering from chronic pain may progress to the point of understanding that change needs to happen, and an appreciation that it will offer them greater pain control. They still do not know how they will change or even how to begin. Regardless, these patients are weighing their alternatives and developing their plans of change. The changes can include adding more favorable coping strategies like relaxation exercises, or adding positive health habits, or abandoning old behaviors that were maladaptive (inactivity, isolation), etc.

The **fourth stage** in the TTM model is **"action."** In this stage, specific change behaviors are identified and a time period and plan are put into place. The work of making change is put into motion.

The **fifth stage** in the TTM model is **"maintenance."** These patients have already established more effective coping strategies in dealing with their chronic pain and have disregarded unfavorable methods of coping. Their daily lives are infused with self-management techniques that better help to manage their chronic pain. This stage makes the patient aware that work must be continued to maintain the changes. It also acknowledges relapse and exacerbations of pain to be challenges. Even so, these patients are reaping the rewards of self-management, and have learned that change is necessary and even advantageous to help control chronic pain successfully.

PSOCQ

The **Pain Stages of Change Questionnaire (PSOCQ)** uses 30 items staged in a self-report fashion to define a patient's readiness for change on a range of four scales. Precontemplation, contemplation, action and maintenance are all considered within these scales, thus including the transtheoretical model of change in the instrument. This instrument can be used as a clinical and/or research tool. More research is needed before health care providers can confidently use this tool as a determinative indicator for clinical decision making. Even so, simply using this self-report tool as a validation of the patient's own admission of readiness to change can be valuable, confirming patient choices empowering them in the formulation and staging of their own treatment plans.

Support Groups

Many **support groups** are facilitated by patients themselves and are often run in volunteer-based organizations as opposed to hospitals, clinics and health care settings. There are even online, chat room and virtual support services available. The purpose of such support groups is to provide social and emotional support and a place where medical information, resources and coping tips can be shared. These groups serve an important purpose, allowing chronic pain patients to feel validated and reducing the sense of isolation they often feel in their suffering. However, these groups can sometimes dispense misinformation and even endorse unfavorable coping strategies. Those support groups that are run on a volunteer basis, in particular, may lack professional medical leadership. Thus, they can often lack specific goals and may counteract specific treatment plans created for individual patients. Therefore, due caution must be exercised with these groups.

Families of Pediatric Chronic Pain Patients

Families of pediatric chronic pain patients may need special assistance in locating support groups suited to their needs. Because pediatric chronic pain clients differ from adults in their needs and abilities to cope, and because of important developmental considerations, not every chronic pain support group will be helpful. Children or adolescents who suffer from chronic pain should not attend support groups aimed at the adult chronic pain patient. The information shared will not be helpful because of the different stages of development they are experiencing. As with adult groups, parents and families must be cautious of the information that is provided, and always validate its accuracy and confirm its cohesiveness with their child's unique treatment plan.

Potential Barriers to Pain Assessment

Potential **barriers to the pain assessment** include:

- Obviously, a **language barrier** may be a potential obstacle to an accurate pain assessment.
- **Culture** can also be a significant barrier to a complete assessment. Different cultures around the world perceive and respond to pain in different ways. Gaining some understanding into the patient's culture without judgment is vital to getting the information needed.
- A patient's **physical and psychological condition** can also be a hurdle, as can certain behavioral considerations. The patient's development level and cognitive ability need to be considered, along with their level on consciousness and ability to be verbal.
- If unable to complete an accurate pain assessment with the patient themselves, solicit others to help gather necessary information.

Barriers to Accurate Pain Assessment Potentially Arising from the Nurse

Successful treatment of pain depends upon quality communication between the patient and the caregiver. While barriers may exist on both sides of this equation, the **nurse** must be aware of any barriers he or she brings to the assessment process. For example, a nurse needs to believe the patient's description of pain in all its facets. Pain must be viewed from the patient's perspective. The nurse must also be able to set aside the burdens of securing, justifying, administering, and documenting analgesics in deference to the patient's needs. Previous experiences of pain for both the nurse and patient and a nurse's understanding of pain grounded in personal and professional beliefs and judgments all play a part in successful communications between the patient and nurse.

Barriers to Pain Management for the Elderly

The **elderly** may underreport pain because of certain persistent biases and beliefs. Among these is the sense that pain is a part of aging or the disease process. Another is the belief that pain is a punishment or penance in their lives, or that it serves to purify and cleanse the soul. The elderly may also believe that pain is normal and expected, and that health care providers will automatically know when they're in pain through medical evaluation and omniscience, and will treat them spontaneously as necessary. Further, elderly patients can feel burdensome as they age and fail to report pain out of a desire to be a "good" patient, or one less troublesome. The cost of treating pain may also become prohibitive for some elderly patients. Related to this, they may not be aware of prescription assistance programs or they're else uncomfortable applying for program benefits they perceive as "indigent welfare".

Barriers to Effectively Managing the Elderly Chronic Pain Patient

The **elderly population** host some unique factors that may negatively affect a health care provider's ability to complete an accurate assessment and render effective treatment.

- Elderly patients may suffer from cognitive impairments making assessments difficult.
- Many elderly patients have dysphasic symptoms or outright aphasia (post stroke, etc.), inhibiting their ability to communicate.
- Health care providers may not be able to accurately distinguish between pain, suffering, and depression in the elderly patient, and thus can easily misinterpret their behaviors.
- Elderly patients are typically on a large number of medications, and polypharmacy interactions can complicate efforts at an accurate assessment.
- Financial constraints may lead to medication non-compliance. However, the health care provider must remain aware of assistance programs and endeavor to ascertain a patient's ability to pay for prescriptions.
- Due to the commitment of time needed to accurately evaluate an elderly chronic pain patient, time constraints may become a barrier to treatment as well.

Risk Assessment of Substance Use

Behaviors That May Raise Concerns About Potential Addiction

There are certain **behaviors** exhibited by individuals that warrant concern about **potential drug addiction**. Selling prescription drugs and forging prescriptions are two such behaviors. An individual may be found stealing or "borrowing" drugs belonging to someone else, or injecting drugs formulated for oral use. Some patients may use non-medical sources to obtain prescription drugs and may also be abusing alcohol or illicit drugs while using prescription medications. Others will use a higher dose than prescribed, or pursue repeated visits to alternate clinicians or emergency departments for the purpose of obtaining prescription drugs. Employment, relationships with family and friends may deteriorate due to the drug-use, and these patients may resist any change in medication therapy.

Risk Assessment Tools for Potential Substance Use
DAST-10

The **DAST-10 screening tool** screens for substance abuse (not including alcohol abuse), defined as the excessive use of over-the-counter medications OR the nonmedical use of drugs. This tool consists of 10 yes or no questions regarding drug use in the last 12 months. Questions are related to drug use, feelings surrounding drug use, the impact of drug use on family, the occurrence of illegal activities surrounding drug use, withdrawal symptoms and medical problems resulting from drug use. Each question is scored 1 or 0 based on yes or no responses and then the degree of the drug abuse problem is based on a total score. Scoring is as follows:

- 0: No problem
- 1-2: Low level problem (monitor/reassess)
- 3-5 Moderate level problem (investigate further)
- 6-8: Substantial problem (intensive assessment required)
- 9-10: Severe problem (intensive assessment required)

NIDA MODIFIED ASSIST DRUG USE SCREENING TOOL

The **NIDA Modified ASSIST Drug Use Screening Tool** begins with a scripted introduction for the interviewer and then starts with a "quick screen" that asks about 4 substance categories: Alcohol, tobacco, prescription drugs for nonmedical reasons, and illegal drugs. The patient responds on a Likert scale regarding frequency of use: Never, once or twice, monthly, weekly, or daily/almost daily. If never is the answer for all questions, the interviewer is advised to continue to encourage abstinence, and the screening is complete. If the patient answers yes (of any quantity to any substance) the interviewer is advised to move on to NIDA-Modified Assist Screen. This consists of 8 questions to clarify the type of substance used, frequency of use, desire/urge to use, problems resulting from use, the impact on responsibilities from this use, whether friends/family have every expressed concern about the use, and failed attempts to stop use. The score is then added up to designate risk:

- 0-3: Lower risk
- 4-26: Moderate risk
- 27+: High risk

CRAFFT SCREENING TOOL

The **CRAFFT Screening Tool** screens for alcohol and drug use, starting with 3 simple yes-or-no questions: Have you drank alcohol, smoked marijuana, or used any other substance to get high in last 12 months (this refers to use in any amount, once or often). If the answer is yes to any of these, the interviewer is then asked to move on to the CRAFFT questions:

- **C**: Have you ever ridden in a CAR driven by someone (including yourself) who was high from alcohol or drugs?
- **R**: Have you ever used drugs/alcohol to help yourself RELAX or feel better about yourself or to fit in?
- **A**: Do you ever use drugs/alcohol when you are ALONE?
- **F**: Do you ever FORGET what you've done when you've used alcohol or drugs?
- **F**: Do your FAMILY/FRIENDS tell you that you should cut down on drug/alcohol use?
- **T**: Have you ever gotten into TROUBLE using drugs/alcohol?

Each YES response is 1 point, and any score >2 is considered positive, requiring additional assessment.

Reassessment of Pain

EVALUATION OF NURSING INTERVENTIONS

Evaluation of specific nursing interventions determines the degree to which they have been successful. The nurse should carefully compare expected outcomes to the actual outcomes of each intervention. Evaluation of the other health care providers to adequately execute appropriate nursing interventions should also occur, as well as determining the patient's ability and opportunity to self-care. In this way the relative contributions of all participants can be examined. The nurse is also responsible for communicating the evaluation findings to the proper health care providers. Reassessments should occur as needed and new, customized interventions should be initiated based upon the ongoing evaluation of outcomes.

Nursing Assessment of Pharmacological Interventions

The **nursing process** is designed to be used on a continuous loop until the resolution of identified problems (i.e., the nursing diagnosis) is achieved. When dealing with chronic pain patients, assessment of pain intensity should be documented before medicine administration to provide a direct correlation of pain resolution once the medication has been given. Reassessing within a short period of time (dependent upon the medication type and route administered) will provide information regarding the efficacy of the medicinal intervention. The outcome will indicate whether or not any changes need to be made to the medication type, regimen, and/or dosage. Prompt action should be taken if the reassessment (evaluation) reveals any inadequacy in pain coverage or if over-sedation occurs. The nursing assessment process then continues in effort to improve outcomes, and/or maintain the status quo.

Nursing Assessment of Non-Pharmacological Interventions

Non-pharmacological interventions can provide adequate pain relief for some patients independently or in conjunction with traditional medicinal therapies. **Reassessing for success with non-medicinal therapies** includes evaluating pain after activities, exercise, massages, heat and cold packs, and position changes. Never assume that a non-pharmacological intervention is exempt from the need for evaluation. Patients may unexpectedly react poorly to environmental changes, position changes, and even massage techniques. Thus, all interventions need to be evaluated, adjusted and revised throughout the nursing process. Evaluation and re-evaluation should continue until satisfactory resolution is achieved (i.e., the goals set by the patient and caregiver have been met and/or are being fully maintained).

Important Terms

Transduction—After peripheral nociceptors are activated by noxious stimuli, the stimulus is changed into electrical impulses. This is change is called transduction.

Transmission—After transduction, an influx of sodium occurs as an outflow of potassium is moving across the neuronal membrane. This quick exchange of electrolytes causes the action potential to progress along the neuronal membrane until it ends in the dorsal horn of the spinal cord. This relay of the transduced impulse is called transmission.

Modulation—Inside the cells of the dorsal horn of the spinal cord, modulation occurs when first phase neurons synapse with second phase neurons. These pain signals can be initiated and amplified by neuropeptides in ascending projection neurons. Concurrently, descending analgesic systems can decrease the nociceptive response.

Perception—Perception occurs when nociceptive signals induce a cerebral cortical recognition or awareness of pain.

Allodynia—Allodynia is a condition where a stimulus that is ordinarily painless is perceived as painful.

Hyperalgesia—Hyperalgesia refers to extreme or exaggerated sensitivity to pain in or around an injured area.

Hyperesthesia—Hyperesthesia is defined as increased sensitivity to many sensory stimuli, such as pain, heat, cold, or touch.

Dysesthesia—Dysesthesia refers to irregular unpleasant and abnormal sensations on or under the skin, often in response to normal stimuli or touch. Feelings of numbness, tingling, prickling, burning or cutting pain on the skin are all included.

Hyperpathia—Hyperpathia describes an exaggerated sense of pain to a known painful stimulus. It differs from allodynia in that the instigating stimulus is painful rather than ordinary.

Raynaud Phenomenon—Raynaud phenomenon is defined as sporadic episodes of pallor trailed by cyanosis, then redness of digits and a return to normal. A person may experience numbness, tingling and burning sensations during the episode. It is usually instigated by exposure to cold or emotional stress.

Radiating—Pain that comes from a localized source and is projected out and into other areas of the body.

Referred—Pain that is perceived as coming from a different location than its actual origin.

Localized—Pain that is perceived in relation to its actual point of origin.

Diffuse—Pain that is scattered or widespread. The patient is not able to pinpoint an origin or central location for the perceived pain.

Temporal—Pain in relation to parameters of time, as when pain is present in the morning but not in the evening, etc.

Hypertonicity—Excess muscular tone or intraocular pressure, seen most often in infants experiencing pain.

Change—Change is the process that leads to alteration in patterns of behavior in an individual or an institution.

Change Agent—Change agent is the person or group who instigates change or who supports others in modifying or changing themselves or an institution or system.

Resistance—Resistance is behavior patterns intended to maintain existing behavior.

Innovation—Innovation is the utilization of new ideas, unique knowledge, skills and experience to derive meaningful benefits. In an organization, this often forms the base of product or service offerings.

Interdependence—Interdependence is a relationship where changes in one faction of the system will cause changes in other parts of the system as well.

Empowerment—Empowerment refers to knowledge and information that enables successful self-direction.

Pseudoaddiction—Drug seeking behavior in an effort to achieve adequate pain relief, not indiscriminate substance abuse.

Physical Dependence—A physiological state in which abrupt discontinuation or dose reduction of an expected opioid, or the administration of an opioid antagonist, will produce a withdrawal response. Physical dependence is expected with the use of opioids on a continuous basis, whether for treatment or recreational use. It does not define addiction.

Tolerance—A need for distinctly increased dosages of substances to achieve intoxication or a desired effect (pain control). Tolerance may also be defined as a significantly decreased effect with continued use of the same amount of a given substance.

Addiction—A loss of control over drug use, as in compulsive drug use and continued use of the drug despite obvious harm. Physical dependence itself does not define addiction.

Interventions

Plan of Care and Interdisciplinary Collaboration

MULTIMODAL PAIN MANAGEMENT

Generally speaking, **multimodal pain management** is defined as the use of multiple (2 or more) methods of pain management to address pain rather than opioids alone. The additional measures of pain management can be other non-opioid analgesic medications, non-analgesic medications (adjuvants), and non-pharmacologic methods. Multimodal pain management is believed to be more effective and to have less side effects than using opioids alone. In order for multimodal pain management to be effective, it must be maintained around the clock to prevent breakthrough pain. Non-opioid pain medications most often include NSAIDS. Non-analgesic medications include adjuvant medications such as anti-convulsants or anti-anxiety medications. Non-pharmacological pain management measures include positioning, environment, distractions, temperature, etc.

INTERDISCIPLINARY INVOLVEMENT IN GOAL SETTING

Chronic pain is a challenging and complex medical problem. There is no single approach to assessment, diagnosis, treatment or evaluation that will solve all of the patient's problems and attend to all of their needs. It is important that additional disciplines (psychosocial, rehabilitative, alternative, nursing, etc.) be brought together when discussing a patient's assessment, diagnosis and treatment plan. When setting goals in an **interdisciplinary** atmosphere, all points of view should be given a voice. Using their different modalities and combining their individual opinions, staff can formulate goals that are appropriate and realistic for the patient. These efforts will enhance treatment plan formulation and success more efficiently than if undertaken alone.

ROLE OF THE PAIN MANAGEMENT PHYSICIAN

Upon accepting a patient into their practice, a **pain management physician** becomes a fully legal, responsible provider. Taking note of existing medical records is appropriate but it is also necessary for a physician to perform and record their own history and physical at the outset. Legally, physicians must accumulate their own information and make their own judgments in accordance with their own professional findings. There is no legal basis for "following another physician's information or orders". The pain management physician should not focus solely on the problem of pain management. Instead he or she should view the patient holistically, looking for interrelated sources of dysfunction that may be undergirding and sustaining the patient's pain. Undiscovered or hidden issues may well be present that could potentially harm the patient or inflate the pain experience.

CONSULTATIVE ROLE OF PAIN MANAGEMENT NURSE

The process of **consultation** includes communication among the health care team in an effort to improve pain management and patient care. As a consultant, the pain management nurse may be asked to directly or indirectly consult on the treatment plan of a patient in pain.

Direct consultation will include an independent assessment of the patient and recommendations for the patient's care derived from that assessment. Indirect consultation would include the pain management nurse offering recommendations or developing a plan of care based upon information supplied by others providing direct care of the patient. The pain management nurse is likely to receive frequent consultation requests regarding the management of a complex pain patient, such as a patient who has undergone surgery who also has concurrent underlying and/or preexisting pain conditions.

Consulting in an indirect capacity may provide the pain management nurse with further opportunities to educate and influence nurses regarding pain management issues. Often nurses hold misconceptions and fears regarding the management of pain in the chemically dependent patient, and others. Education can help to dispel the myths associated with their care and help the nursing staff create an appropriate, successful pain management plan.

As a consultant, the pain management nurse should develop a formal evaluation process by which to respond to requests. Educational goals may even include having direct care nurses report identified outcomes and progress to the pain management nurse, along with their reassessment of objectives, continuing concerns, and successes.

Pharmacological Treatment

PHARMACOKINETICS

When drugs are administered for pain management, the **pharmacokinetics** of different routes of administration are evaluated by four indices:

- **Absorption:** How and where the drug is absorbed most effectively.
- **Distribution:** How the drug is distributed by differing routes of administration.
- **Metabolism:** Where and how a drug is metabolized in the body. This is important in choosing the drug and dosage for treatment.
- **Elimination:** How a drug is eliminated from the body. Dependent upon a patient's body function, different drugs may be chosen.

The development and use of controlled-release dosages of certain drugs has added another element to be taken into consideration when evaluating the pharmacokinetics of various drugs.

DISTRIBUTION OF OPIOID MEDICATIONS

The **distribution** of a drug refers to its pattern of travel from the blood stream to differing tissues of the body and its intended site of action. The determining factors in the distribution of opioid medications are their ability to bind to plasma protein and their degree of lipophilicity. Morphine is 30 to 35 percent bound to plasma proteins and is hydrophilic, thus morphine does not linger in body tissue for an extended period of time. Fentanyl on the other hand is 80 to 85 percent bound to plasma proteins and is quite lipophilic. Fat tissue is a reservoir for fentanyl, redistributing the drug slowly into circulation.

ELIMINATION OF MEDICATIONS

The process of drug **elimination** is defined as the excretion of drugs, including the active and inactive metabolites, from the body. Common routs of elimination are through the kidneys, lungs (if drugs are administered into the respiratory system, they are more likely to be eliminated there), sweat and salivary glands, intestinal tract (excretion) as well as mammary glands (i.e., breast milk). Patients with compromised kidney function who are also on hemodialysis will have some medications eliminated through the dialysis process. Opioids are excreted by the kidneys at a rate of nearly 90 percent. Both parent drugs and metabolites are excreted in this manner. Elimination in fecal matter accounts for only 10 percent of the elimination of opioid medications.

Metabolism of Hydrophilic Drugs

The chemical reactions involved in the biotransformation of medications into water soluble compounds (metabolites) are called drug **metabolism**. These water-soluble compounds are ionized to an acceptable pH and excreted by the kidneys. The liver, intestinal mucosa, central nervous system, kidneys, skin, lungs and placenta are all sites of drug metabolism. The kidney metabolizes and excretes many opioids directly, with those that haven't been easily eliminated by the kidneys being metabolized further by the liver into more water-soluble metabolites. The liver also metabolizes other opioids (particularly those that are lipophilic. Toxicity is a concern with opioid treatment because an accumulation of metabolites and/or the parent compounds can sometimes occur, particularly in patients with decreased kidney and/or liver function.

The WHO's Principles Regarding Opioid Use and the Analgesic Ladder

The **WHO Recommended Opioid Use Principles** are:

1. Use oral or other noninvasive routes whenever possible.
2. Individualize doses by titrating to response.
3. Select analgesics according to needs as described on the analgesic ladder.
4. Maintain effective drug levels in the body as long as there is a noxious stimulus.
5. Use indicated adjuvant medications.

The World Health Organization (WHO) has developed a three-step ladder for cancer pain treatment. It is to be used to help lessen or eliminate cancer pain. The steps are as follows: Step one: use non-opioid treatment with or without an adjuvant. Step two: if pain increases or is persistent, administer an opioid for mild to moderate pain plus a non-opioid and with or without an adjuvant. Step three: if pain continues or increases, opioids to control moderate to severe pain should be administered along with a non-opioid and with or without an adjuvant.

Classifications of Drugs with Potential for Abuse

In **1970 The Comprehensive Drug Abuse Prevention and Control Act** was passed, classifying drugs with the potential for being abused according to 5 subgroups. Schedule V are drugs that are believed to hold little potential for abuse. Schedule I drugs carry the highest risk of potential abuse. Physicians, pharmacists and nurses can all be held legally responsible for medicinal treatments. Pharmacists are held to different legal standards in different states, but are federally mandated to provide a check and balance for doctors prescribing opioids. Nurses can be held legally responsible for both inadequate and/or inappropriate opioid therapy administration.

Principles of Analgesic Management

The following are **basic principles of analgesic management**:

- **Titration and rotation** – In medicine, titration refers to small and/or gradual changes in doses of prescribed medication to achieve the necessary effect. Titration of analgesia medication is used to find an optimal dose for each individual patient. Pain control and severity of side effects should both be considered when titrating doses. Rotating (alternating) doses of medications that can be taken concurrently (e.g., acetaminophen and ibuprofen) can provide improved pain control as compared to either medication used continuously or alone.
- **Scheduled dosing** – Administering medication on a schedule is required for pain that is anticipated to last longer than twelve to twenty-four hours. This will help avoid any recurrence of pain and ultimately reduces the total dosage required to maintain pain control. Once acute pain begins to resolve a "prn" (as needed) schedule can be adopted.

The following are additional **principles of analgesic management:**

- **Patient safety** – is always the foremost concern. Before medicating any individual, triple check to verify allergies, drug-to-drug interactions and diagnosis in relation to any expected adverse side effects.
- **Match the drug to pain intensity** – choose the drug that provides the fewest side effects or drug-to-drug interactions, while maintaining adequate pain coverage.
- **Individualized regimen** – recognize that each individual will absorb, metabolize and eliminate drugs to different degrees. Side effects will also be different and will affect individuals in uniquely varying ways. Each patient should also receive an individualized treatment plan for analgesia.
- **Equianalgesic** – the dose of one type of analgesic drug that is equivalent in pain-relieving ability to a differing analgesia. Side effects may make some drugs prohibitive. Because various analgesic medications have different potencies, it is important to know at which dosages they have equal potential to fight pain.
- **Least invasive route of administration first:** Always choose the route that is least invasive, if it can be equally effective. Oral opioids produce similar and adequate results in comparison to parenteral routes that are more invasive, have greater side effects, can inflict more pain and carry the potential for increased difficulties (patency of IV, infection, etc.).
- **Multimodal approach:** Draw from all methods of pain control at one's disposal, as this has the greatest potential to successfully decrease a patient's pain. Utilize environmental considerations, spiritual care, cognitive-behavioral therapy, thermal modalities, massage, positioning, exercise, range-of-motion exercises, etc., to compliment pharmaceutical analgesic methods.

Opioid Analgesics

TRANSDERMAL ADMINISTRATION OF OPIOID MEDICATIONS

Transdermal opioid administration is useful in patients who are suffering from gastrointestinal issues that would affect oral administration. This method of administration is also often used with non-opioid and adjuvant analgesics. Transdermal opioid administration should not be used in patients who have never before used opioids, or for rapid escalation. Therapeutic levels are reached twelve hours after placement of a patch and last for forty-eight to seventy-two hours. Patients should also be given a method to manage breakthrough pain, as the transdermal route does not allow for rapid dose increases. Be sure to educate the patient on the risk of constipation. Emphasize that the patch placement site should be rotated. Further, the skin should always be dry and intact before patch placement, and a transparent dressing may be needed to maintain patch contact with the skin. Finally, patients should also be advised about what to do if the patch falls off, as well as being informed about possible side effects and the signs and symptoms of withdrawal.

FENTANYL ADMINISTERED THROUGH TRANSDERMAL AND TRANSMUCOSAL ROUTES

When considering transdermal and transmucosal administration, opioids that are lipophilic (e.g., fentanyl) pass more readily through these routes than medications that are hydrophilic (e.g., morphine). **Transdermal fentanyl patches** release medication into the subcutaneous fat under the skin. This area acts as a drug reservoir; thus, the medication is released slowly over two to three days. Serum levels of the medication rise slowly, somewhere around 15-20 hours and may continue for 12 to 24 hours post-patch removal. This drug is ideal for patients with established, predictable opioid needs. **Transmucosal administration** will provide onset of analgesia in 5 to 10 minutes with a peak effect in 20 to 40 minutes. These preparations are used for preoperative and pre-procedural pain and can be very helpful with breakthrough cancer pain.

ORAL ADMINISTRATION OF OPIOID MEDICATIONS

Systemic opioid administration is most often achieved by **oral administration.** Within twenty to ninety minutes, the medication is at its peak, lasting from three to six hours. This route is the easiest and offers the most choices: more drugs come in oral form, and there are extended (controlled) release preparations. Patients with hepatic irregularities and/or renal issues need to consider an opioid that does not accumulate metabolites. If gastrointestinal tract issues exist, resulting in absorption irregularities, non-oral opioids need to be considered as the drug will not be absorbed properly, leading to inadequate pain control and possible toxicity. Both opioids and adjuvant therapies can be given orally, and used together. Patients should be educated on possible bowel complications (constipation), signs and symptoms of opioid withdrawal, dose escalation (due to worsening pain and/or tolerance development), and side effects.

RECTAL AND TOPICAL ADMINISTRATION OF OPIOID MEDICATIONS

There are many advantages to **rectal drug administration**. The rectal surface is highly vascularized, and thus drugs are readily absorbed. The blood that perfuses the rectum bypasses the liver, so medications administered rectally will bypass first-pass hepatic metabolism. Drugs administered rectally also absorb at a slow and steady pace. When the gastrointestinal tract is irritated or not functioning properly, rectal administration may well be preferred. However, erratic absorption is possible if bowel contents interfere, or if the medications are unexpectedly expelled through a bowel movement. Thus, a preparatory enema may sometimes be helpful. If a patient suffers from rectal irritation, bleeding, diarrhea or hemorrhoids, the rectal route is not ideal.

Topical medication administration is reserved for medications not suitable for injection because they may infect or irritate the tissue. Topical medications come in cream, gel or ointment preparations, and patients should be educated on safe and effective application of the medications.

ABSORPTION OF MORPHINE ADMINISTERED ORALLY AND RECTALLY

Morphine and other opioids are easily absorbed from the GI tract, whether by oral or rectal administration. Both of these methods of administration are convenient, simple and inexpensive, and often less traumatic for patients than intravenous administration of a drug. Opioids taken orally will pass through the liver before entering the blood stream and causing a systemic analgesic effect. Thus, stronger doses of morphine will be needed to accommodate this first-line metabolism process. Onset of pain control will occur about 20 to 40 minutes after administration of most immediate-release oral opioids. Peak analgesia requires an elapse of 45 to 60 minutes, although the exact time is dependent on the immediate form of the drug. Rectal administration of opioids will not be subject to first-pass metabolism, and doses should be adjusted accordingly.

SUBCUTANEOUS INFUSION OF OPIOID MEDICATIONS

Oral opioid administration is preferred, but there are cases when patients cannot tolerate oral preparations. Before turning to intravenous administration, which is invasive and may not be advantageous or dependable, **subcutaneous infusion** should be considered. Both intravenous and subcutaneous administrations provide similar serum levels of the opioid for the first 24 hours and drop off after 48 hours. With subcutaneous infusion the patient should achieve a steady-state of analgesia, with the option of using both continuous infusion and bolus administration. Subcutaneous infusion is less invasive than IV therapy and anti-emetics can be administered at the same time. In comparing subcutaneous injections, intramuscular injections and subcutaneous infusions, the time frames for therapeutic levels are comparable and possibly less invasive.

ABSORPTION OF OPIOID MEDICATIONS ADMINISTERED BY INTRAVENOUS ROUTES

Intravenous administration of opioid medications will provide, in theory, 100% bioavailability. Subcutaneous and intramuscular injections provide similar drug levels to those administered by IV infusion. Drugs that are more lipophilic (Fentanyl) will act quickly after injection in comparison to those opioids that are hydrophilic (morphine).

Subcutaneous and intramuscular administration will be somewhat delayed due to absorption, but ultimately will provide similar blood serum levels at similar times. Intramuscular (IM) administration is not ideal as it can cause tissue damage and significant pain, and because absorption of these medications via IM administration can be unpredictable (lipophilicity is a major contributing factor).

INTRASPINAL ADMINISTRATION OF OPIOID MEDICATIONS

Intraspinal administration of opioids is the administration of such medications into the epidural or intrathecal space. Opioids administered via this route do not cause marked sedative effects, as compared to IV, subcutaneous and intramuscular administration. They do, however, cause respiratory depression, nausea, urinary retention and itching. Further, sedation will still occur at higher dosages. Postural hypotension may also occur, as well as numbness.

Opioids administered into the **epidural space** will diffuse through the dura and bind at the dorsal horn of the spinal cord. Fentanyl is a lipophilic opioid and thus will diffuse rapidly through the dura providing a narrower range of analgesia. Morphine, by comparison, is hydrophilic and diffuses slowly through the dura, thus creating a wider analgesic window.

PCA

Patient controlled analgesia (PCA) is an intravenous administration controlled by the patient. It provides for both intermittent and continuous pain control. It is used widely for postoperative patients, patients with traumatic injuries, acute medical episodes, and pain experienced during procedures. It can be used with a bolus dose that is patient initiated, or with a continuous infusion and patient controlled bolus dose.

BOLUS DOSE INFUSION COUPLED WITH CONTINUOUS INFUSION

Bolus dose infusion coupled with continuous infusion (a constant low-dose infusion of an opioid given through the PCA device) will help preserve a continuously effective opioid concentration. With a bolus dose alone, the patient may be affected by interim opioid concentrations that are not therapeutic; but when the continuous infusion is employed, that is not likely. With this approach the patient can even fall asleep and still get the continuous dosage of opioid needed to largely control their pain. Continuous infusion is also called a basal rate or background infusion. However, continuous infusion may cause an accumulation of the opioid. Thus, these patients need regularly scheduled assessments for respiratory depression and changes in mental status. The side effects of opioids may also be felt more significantly when given through a continuous infusion. These include vomiting, itching, urinary retention, sedation and respiratory depression.

BOLUS DOSE ADMINISTRATION OF PAIN MEDICATION

Patient-controlled bolus dose opioid infusion is used for "on demand" pain control in a single dose (i.e., for break-through pain). It is delivered through a PCA device that is triggered when the patient presses a button kept at the bedside. There is a lock-out period to ensure safe timing of doses (i.e., the patient can push the button as often as they like but will only receive medication when the scheduled amount of time has passed). This method avoids the ups and downs that are common between analgesia, sedation and pain; it also minimizes the risk of opioids accumulating in the blood stream. The PCA patient may run into trouble when they are sleeping (i.e., they will not receive the bolus dose if the button is not pushed).

Teaching Patients Using PCA

Patient-controlled analgesia (PCA) is commonly used pre-procedurally as well as post-operatively. Patients who will be using a PCA should be taught how to use the device before surgery or procedures begin. Staff should explain when to push the button as well as the time lock out function that will prevent inadvertent over dosing, as the patient may be particularly concerned with receiving medication too often. Specifically discuss with the patient who is allowed to push the button. Discuss parameters for communicating with the nurse regarding any unsatisfactory results (i.e., feeling too sedated, bothered by side effects such as itching, vomiting, and inability to void, etc.) Be sure to set goals for the patient's pain control, keeping in mind that complete pain control is probably not attainable. Lastly, educate the patient regarding opioid addiction and the function of pain in recovery. Encourage them to use the PCA as needed, emphasizing that it is safe and appropriate for their circumstance.

Joint Commission's Guidelines for Opioid Administration Documentation

Every accredited agency must follow the **Joint Commission's guidelines for opioid administration documentation.** Although they may have individualized protocols, these must still fall within the guidelines. Documentation must show that each patient is assessed for pain on admission and on regular, continuing intervals during a hospitalization. The reported pain value should be documented as well as what was given, when, and by what route. Pain relief efficacy needs to be evaluated after an appropriate lapse of time (dependent on route of administration and peak time of the administered drug) and also documented. This process must continue until realistic goals of pain control have been reached. Joint Commission guidelines may change, as well as agency policy. Thus, it is up to the nurse to stay regularly apprised of all required documentation for opioid administration.

Proper Documentation of Opioid Administration

A nurse has a responsibility to **document opioid administration** accurately. The amount and dosage of the opioid should be duly recorded as well as the route by which it was administered. Documentation of the dose administered along with the observed or reported response to that dose is also required. Opioids that are being administered via an infusion device should be documented cumulatively every three to four hours. Protocols for the waste (discarding) of opioids should be established and carefully followed. Special considerations should be made for opioids that are contained in infusion bags, used in home health care settings, or those used in settings where known drug abuse is a problem. Some facilities may also require a follow up pain assessment in the case of providing PRN pain medication to a patient. Generally, this re-assessment occurs one hour after the medication has been administered, using whatever pain scale the patient is able to demonstrate. Refer to facility procedures and protocols regarding pain reassessment post-PRN pain medication administration.

Non-Opioid Analgesics

NSAIDs

Nonsteroidal anti-inflammatory drugs (NSAIDs) are the most commonly used of all drugs. Pain and stiffness are reduced, and improved function is realized for those with in osteoarthritis, rheumatoid and other forms of arthritis when NSAIDs are used. They reduce both swelling and pain. NSAIDs are absorbed well after oral administration, although these rates may vary with patients who are affected by gastrointestinal blood flow and/or motility issues. NSAIDs are more than 95 percent bound to serum albumin and thus caution must be taken to avoid increases of the free component of NSAID in serum levels. Particular care should be taken if patients experience decreasing serum albumin levels, or when taking other highly-protein bound medications. These drugs are metabolized by the liver, primarily, and excreted in the urine.

SIDE EFFECTS

Nonsteroidal anti-inflammatory drugs are associated with the following side effects:

- **Gastrointestinal Symptoms:** Dyspepsia, nausea, vomiting, diarrhea or constipation, reflux (burning in the chest, possibly tasting gastric juices in the mouth), and ulcerations (bleeding).
- **Renal Symptoms:** Lower extremity edema due to sodium and water retention, secondary to renal dysfunction.
- **Hematological Symptoms:** Increased bleeding and/or bruising (platelet aggregation is affected by NSAID use, as is bleeding time).
- **Central Nervous System Symptoms:** Sedation, confusion, headache, depression and psychosis.
- **Hepatic Symptoms:** Elevated hepatic lab values.
- **Pulmonary Symptoms:** Increased asthma symptoms.

ACETAMINOPHEN

To inhibit pain and decrease fever, **acetaminophen** inhibits prostaglandin synthetase in the central nervous system. It is not an effective anti-inflammatory agent, but it is highly effective with mild to moderate nociceptive pain. While acetaminophen is widely used and available over-the-counter, it does have the potential to create hepatic dysfunction. The dosage of acetaminophen should be specifically limited if the patient drinks alcohol, and periodic liver function tests are advisable with continuous use. Symptoms of possible acute toxicity include but are not limited to nausea, vomiting and abdominal pain. Acetaminophen may mask infection and there are potential drug interactions that must be guarded against by health care providers. Even so, the frequency of adverse side effects is low. Acetaminophen is often used as an adjuvant therapy or it can be effective alone.

TOPICAL ANALGESIC AGENTS

Topical agents are gels, creams, lotions or patches applied directly where the pain is originating. They are particularly advantageous because they do not increase serum levels of the prescribed medication, leading to lower drug to drug interactions as well as fewer side effects. The time from administration to helpful effect is reportedly much shorter than with oral administration, as topical administration skips the need for absorption and provides less need for titration of dose. Lidocaine cream 2.5% has been shown to be more effective in neuropathic pain than the oral counterparts. Other topical preparations may be used with arthritis. These drugs work by decreasing or preventing an increase in the permeability of excitable membranes to sodium, causing a block in nerve conduction. Typically, side effects related to topical administration of analgesic are limited to rash and dermatitis at the site of application.

ANTIDEPRESSANTS

Antidepressants are believed to have an analgesic component that is separate from their known antidepressant affects. Chronic pain conditions, particularly those with a neuropathic component, are likely to benefit from inclusion of antidepressants in the treatment plan. Antidepressants are divided into several categories. Tricyclic antidepressants, selective serotonin reuptake inhibitors, and atypical antidepressants all may be beneficial to the chronic pain patient. Certain tricyclic antidepressants are used more often than others, to limit various side effects. Patients may need a baseline or updated electrocardiogram before beginning therapy with a tricyclic antidepressant because of possible cardiac side effects. Elderly patients may not tolerate the typical anticholinergic effects of tricyclic medications.

ATYPICAL ANTIDEPRESSANTS

Atypical antidepressants include trazodone, nefazodone, bupropion and venlafaxine.

- **Trazodone** selectively inhibits the reuptake of serotonin and is well absorbed orally. It is metabolized nearly completely by the liver and is eliminated through the urine. The drug is moderately sedating and thus is frequently used in instances of depression combined with mild insomnia. There appears to be little analgesic effect.
- **Nefazodone** inhibits the reuptake of both serotonin and norepinephrine. There are fewer anti-cholinergic side effects and it is less likely to cause sexual dysfunction. Nefazodone may well have analgesic properties.
- **Bupropion's** pharmacologic processes remain unclear. Analgesic effects are minimal, but it is effective as an aide in smoking cessation. This drug has less anticholinergic side effects than many other antidepressants.

TRICYCLIC ANTIDEPRESSANTS

After oral administration, **tricyclic antidepressants** soon achieve good bioavailability. However, when orally administered they are metabolized extensively on hepatic first-pass, and are exceedingly protein bound. Being highly lipophilic their distribution also differs greatly with body composition. While the therapeutic serum level of tricyclic antidepressants in treatment for depression is known, less is known about levels necessary for a therapeutic analgesic effect. It is generally thought to be less than the level needed to-treat depression, but this remains unproven. Tricyclic antidepressants work by inhibiting presynaptic neuronal reuptake of norepinephrine and serotonin. Side effects include: Anticholinergic symptoms (dry mouth, constipation, blurred vision, and urinary retention), sedation, orthostatic hypotension, lower seizure threshold, increased appetite and weight gain, tachycardia, arrhythmias and hypotension.

SSRIs

Selective serotonin reuptake inhibitors (SSRIs) work by inhibiting presynaptic neuronal uptake of serotonin. SSRIs include: fluoxetine, paroxetine, sertraline, citalopram and fluvoxamine. These drugs are useful only for adjuvant analgesia, as their main mechanism of action (serotonin reuptake blockade) is ineffective in pain management alone. They are recommended for use in patients affected by headaches, diabetic neuropathy, chronic pelvic pain and fibrositis. Common SSRI side effects include: insomnia, agitation, anxiety, tremor, sexual dysfunction and gastrointestinal distress. Fluoxetine may also cause significant weight loss; thus, caution is warranted in use with underweight depressed patients. These drugs are not recommended as primary tools for chronic pain treatment. However, using these drugs in end-stage disease may be very helpful with pain and depression.

ANTICONVULSANTS

Anticonvulsants include: phenytoin, carbamazepine, valproic acid, clonazepam, gabapentin and lamotrigine. Anticonvulsants are used as effective analgesics for chronic neuropathic pain, particularly when the pain is lancinating and burning in nature. These drugs have been researched and proven highly effective against trigeminal neuralgia, glossopharyngeal neuralgia, neuralgia post therapy and diabetic neuropathies and possible cancer pain with a neuropathic component.

Carbamazepine is typically the drug of choice. Carbamazepine is chemically similar to a tricyclic antidepressant. Absorption is slow and inconsistent with oral administration. The drug is metabolized in the liver and excreted in the urine. Neuropathic pain may involve spontaneous electrical activity involving ectopic foci of dysfunctional sodium channels in injured nerves. Carbamazepine slows the rate of recovery of inactivated sodium channels, which may stabilize of neuronal membranes. Side effects include: sedation, dizziness, ataxia, confusion, headache and constipation.

LOCAL ANESTHETICS

Local anesthetics are thought to be effective for the treatment of chronic pain if the pain is neuropathic in origin. Commonly used drugs include: intravenous lidocaine and oral preparations such as mexiletine and tocainide. Tocainide has a high risk of toxicity, so mexiletine is the oral drug of choice. Typically, these drugs would be used after trials of antidepressants and anticonvulsants have failed. These drugs block the conduction of nerve impulses by decreasing or preventing permeability of excitable membranes to sodium. Lidocaine is poorly absorbed orally, and sixty to seventy percent of the drug is metabolized by the liver before it ever reaches systemic circulation. However, Mexiletine has a high rate of oral absorption, and only 10 percent of the drug is not metabolized by the time it reaches the kidneys.

Common **lidocaine** side effects are: lightheadedness and dizziness, tinnitus, vertigo, blurred vision and altered taste. Seizures can occur at higher doses and cardiac side effects (which may occur at even higher serum levels) include hypotension, bradycardia, and cardiovascular collapse, which can lead to cardiac arrest.

Mexiletine side effects include: nausea, vomiting, diplopia and tremor. Mexiletine can cause increased atrioventricular conduction time, so it is contraindicated for patients with a second- or third-degree heart block. Taking mexiletine with food may help to decrease the nausea and vomiting. Lidocaine infusions should be followed with mexiletine to provide the best pain management results. Cardiac monitoring should be completed before lidocaine is infused. Mexiletine doses should be increased slowly to help dissipate side effects such as tremor and diplopia.

CORTICOSTEROIDS

Corticosteroids are used as an adjuvant treatment when inflammation or massive edema is the origin of pain. These drugs inhibit phospholipase activity, and then prostaglandin synthesis. They may also reduce axonal sprouting and neurokinin levels in the sensory fibers near injured tissues. Axons that are regenerating in neuromas discharge naturally or with minimal tactile stimulation because there are sensitive sodium channels involved. It appears that corticosteroids reduce neuroma discharge. Corticosteroids run high risks of toxicity and other side effects when they are used long-term. Side effects include: fluid retention, electrolyte disturbances, hypertension, proximal myopathy, osteoporosis and aseptic necrosis, insomnia, psychosis, gastritis, hyperglycemia and impaired cellular immunity. Corticosteroids may also cause elevated mood, antiemesis and appetite stimulation. However, these effects may decrease as the drug is taken longer.

Adjuvant Medications

Adjuvant pain medications are medications that are not primarily utilized to treat pain but, when used in conjunction with pain medication, can enhance pain management. Examples of adjuvant pain medications include the following:

- **Anticonvulsants**: May be effective for nerve pain.
- **Antidepressants**: Have been noted for helping with nerve pain, headaches and RA.
- **Sedatives**: Because pain can interrupt sleep, and sleep is important in healing, sedatives allow for sleep in a patient too uncomfortable to sleep otherwise, and can lead to healing and pain alleviation.
- **Muscle relaxers**: Effective for acute nerve pain that has resulted in the tensing of muscles, but not ideal for chronic pain.
- **Anti-anxiety medications**: Because anxiety can worsen pain, managing anxiety can help treat pain in a secondary fashion.

Herbal Medicine

Herbal medicine is often looked upon as inferior to the synthesized compounds we use as medicine today. However, this belief is held primarily in mainstream America, as Europeans use herbal treatments fervently and have produced a large body of research and information in phytomedicine, or herbal remedies. In truth, many of the drugs we use today are derived directly from plant sources. For example, opioid analgesics are derivatives of the poppy plant and have simply been refined to remove impurities. Digoxin (sold under brand names such as Crystodigin and Lanoxin) is derived from the digitalis, or Foxglove, plant family, and has been used for cardiac treatments since at least 1785. Even so, more research is often believed to be needed to secure herbal remedies a place in modern Western medicine, along with federal regulations regarding the safety and efficacy of such treatments.

Medication Safety and Misuse

Common Myths and Misconceptions Regarding Opioids
Addiction and Dependence

It is important to note that most patients in pain are seeking comfort and relief, not seeking to get high. Research shows that **opioid addiction originating from therapeutic use** is extremely rare. Patients who are opioid-naïve are actually more apt to experience dysphoria than euphoria when undergoing opioid therapy. Drug-seeking behavior in patients with severe and excruciating pain does not in and of itself suggest addiction. Patients who are in severe pain may become obsessed with finding relief (i.e. opioid therapy) rather than fixated the drug itself. This need is termed **pseudoaddiction**. Situational drug dependence, sufficient to produce at least some withdrawal symptoms, is a predictable occurrence in patients who take opioids for more than a few days. Dosages should be leveled off slowly to minimize the withdrawal effects. However, neither fear of dependence nor fear of addiction should be barriers to the proper use of opioid therapy in treating pain.

Multiple Pain Complaints

Many health care providers mistakenly assume that a patient is becoming abusive of the opioid treatment when new pain complaints arise. However, patients with severe and chronic pain are often afflicted with pain from multiple causes. In addition, greater pain can often mask pain of less intensity until the greater pain is controlled. Thus, it is important to remember that defining pain's existence is solely up to the patient.

Saving Opioid Therapy Until Truly Needed

Many providers also are under the false assumption that opioids should be saved for the management of more severe pain as a disease or condition progresses, so that their efficacy is not diminished by use too early. However, opioid dosages can continually be increased to clinically safe doses and thereby retain effectiveness.

Effectiveness for All Types of Pain

Opioids are effective as pain control therapy for most nociceptive pain and a great deal of neuropathic pain. However, it is a misconception that opioids are effective for all types of pain. There are some types of pain that are indeed opioid-responsive but where the pain may be better treated by other analgesics, or where other treatments should at least be considered first (i.e., constipation pain, etc.).

Parenterally Administered Opioids Are More Effective Than Their Oral Counterparts

Parenteral and oral routes of administration are equally effective, as are other noninvasive routes as well. However, many patients believe parenteral medications are a sign that their disease is progressing. This may cause unneeded stress and anxiety, and should be addressed as needed. Finally, potency is not equivalent to efficacy. Some drugs need stronger doses to reach the same clinical outcome as other drugs, yet both have may have the same efficacy, albeit different potencies.

Safe Driving and Opiophobia

As opioid therapy is initiated or dosages are increased, noticeable impairments in judgment and psychomotor function are apt to occur. However, within a week's time of consistent use it is normal to see these side effects resolve. There is formal research that supports this observation. Thus, a patient can typically go about their daily activities, including driving, once a consistent dose has been established and symptoms of opioid induced impairment are no longer noted. Even so, these same patients should not drive any time their dosage is being altered, until they have no signs of impairment for a full week.

Opiophobia is defined as the irrational and unsubstantiated fear that appropriate use of opioids will cause addiction.

Predisposing Conservative Incremental Dose Increases of Opioids During Pain Treatment

Fears regarding the safety of opioid therapy in chronic pain cause many providers to use conservative dose increases when titrating opioid medications. This practice can lead to unsuccessful pain control with opioid therapy. When a patient knows they are receiving an increased dose of opioid medication but their pain does not respond accordingly, anxiety and stress can increase leading to increased pain perceptions. Thus, the dose should be increased substantially, sufficient to achieve the reported response. An appropriate increment is typically 50 percent of the last dose, regardless of the previous dose amount. If sedation initially occurs at a higher dose, it may well be advantageous to the patient who is likely anxious and unable to sleep.

Additional Concerns and Fears Regarding Pain Management

Health care providers have the important task of assessing a patient's pain and acting on therapeutic interventions to help alleviate that pain. Such a daunting task does not come without **provider fears and concerns regarding proper care.** Health care providers can be fearful of being fooled or tricked into administering medication for pain that the patient is not actually experiencing. Also, the health care provider may have the fear of investigation and loss of licensure (with the resulting loss of their career and livelihood) for inappropriate administration of opioids. There are many regulations aimed at preventing drug abuse and inappropriate drug administration that can paralyze a health care provider when the parameters of a specific case are not clear.

Opioid Tolerance

Tolerance, including a reduction in respiratory depression and other components of central nervous system depression, can develop within five to seven days of uninterrupted opioid use. Patients experiencing such accommodation are termed opioid tolerant. However, tolerance to the constipation that accompanies opioid use does not occur, as peristalsis is inhibited in the colon by activated opioid receptors. Therefore, laxatives are needed to stimulate colonic emptying and to reduce the risk of severe constipation and fecal impaction. Stool softeners alone will not work. Finding a therapeutic opioid dose for optimum pain control will take time. Titrating the dose over several days up to a week is expected. Once a therapeutic dose is achieved, there is usually no more need to further titrate the dosage, unless added factors such as new pathologies, drug interactions, or new activities or exercises are commenced with less pain, or if noncompliance becomes an issue.

Tolerance, Physical Dependence, and Addiction

Tolerance and physical dependence are considered pharmacologic properties of opioids and are expected, clinical reactions to opioid therapy. Tolerance is a need for an increased dosage to provide previously established analgesia at lower opioid levels. Physical dependence is what happens when drug therapy is abruptly stopped, or when an antagonist is administered, reversing the effects of the opioid immediately, and it results in a withdrawal process. Dependence is expected in all patients who use opioid medications. Neither tolerance nor physical dependence indicates addiction by themselves. Addiction is the compulsive use of a substance despite physical, psychological, or social harm, including continued use despite the harmful effects. Tolerance and physical dependence, including the ensuing withdrawal symptoms, are not indicators of addiction by themselves.

Tolerance Related to Opioid Therapy

Tolerance is considered a physiologic response and should be expected in patients who are exposed to opioid therapy over a long period of time. Tolerance by itself is not an indicator of addiction, and patients experiencing tolerance should be given a higher dose of medication to control their pain, or the opioid should be changed. Some patients will respond to a different opioid with maximum analgesic affect. This suggests that cross-tolerance between opioids is not complete. Because cross-tolerance is not prohibitive, new opioids should be given at smaller doses and titrated to successful analgesia levels. Tolerance can also be developed for opioid side effects (nausea, pruritus, etc.) over varying periods of time.

Tolerance and Palliative Care

In nearly all cases the argument for increasing the opioid dose is valid, as tolerance in and of itself does not define addiction and tolerance is to be expected in the administration of opioids. Generally, if a patient's disease process is stable a clinically significant dosage can be agreed upon long term. However, in the case of a patient receiving **palliative care** the need for increasing dosages of opioid therapy can likely be attributed to progressing disease and appropriate increases in opioid therapy should be administered. These changes can be quite large, sometimes as much as twenty-fold increases.

Opioid Withdrawal

Opioid withdrawal most often begins with the least severe symptoms first, followed by more severe consequences. Withdrawal can occur with even minimal opioid use. Sudden discontinuation of any opioid or the use of an opioid antagonist will incite withdrawal symptoms. Shorter acting opioids such as morphine or hydromorphone are more likely to cause withdrawal symptoms than longer acting and/or transdermally administered agents such as fentanyl or methadone. When withdrawing the patient will become increasingly irritable, restless and anxious, and may yawn frequently. They may also suffer from insomnia, sweating, rhinorrhea and lacrimation. As withdrawal progresses gooseflesh, dilated pupils, tremor, chills, anorexia, muscle cramps, nausea, vomiting, abdominal pain, diarrhea, agitation, fever, tachycardia and other clinical manifestations may appear, as evidence of a heightened sympathetic system.

PREVENTING OR REVERSING SYMPTOMS

If opioid withdrawal is to be avoided, slow, systematic diminishing doses of the opioid should be continued over a period of time. Reducing the medication at a rate of 15 to 20 percent every 24-48 hours can usually prevent most if not all withdrawal symptoms. If withdrawal has already begun, reintroducing the opioid at smaller dosages (25 to 40 percent of the previous day's dosage) can usually reverse the withdrawal symptoms the patient is suffering from. To help prevent sleep disturbances such as insomnia, which is often associated with opioid withdrawal, eliminate the bedtime dosing last, at the very end of the weaning process. Sympatholytics can be used to decrease the sympathetic hyperactivity that is also common during opioid withdrawal. Clonidine and beta blockers are both effective sympatholytics. However, such drugs cause hypotension and thus due caution must be exercised.

Side Effects of Pharmacologic Interventions

ASSESSMENT OF SIDE EFFECTS DURING PAIN MANAGEMENT THERAPY

Because analgesics (including opioids, non-steroidal anti-inflammatory drugs, acetaminophen, anti-epileptics, anti-depressants, corticosteroids and others) have a vast array of side effects it is important to know the **pharmacokinetics** of each drug as well as the **potential side effects** and drug or disease/condition interactions. Often, particularly with opioids, the side effects can be managed simply by titrating the dose to a lower level slowly, so as to retain analgesia. Other times the drugs may need to be discontinued when poor or even life-threatening side effects result. Knowing the drugs being administered, their side effects, drug-to-drug interactions and contraindicated diagnoses is vital to the safety of patients.

SIDE EFFECTS RELATED TO OPIOID THERAPY
RESPIRATORY DEPRESSION

Respiratory depression is a serious side effect resulting from systemic opioid therapy. Whether the drug is given orally, parenterally or by any other route, respiratory depression is possible. Respiratory depression is always preceded by subtle changes in mental status (confusion, sedation, etc.) that could easily be seen as side effects of the pain itself and/or as related to an ensuing painful event. Thus, mental status should be assessed every hour so that respiratory depression can be promptly identified. At onset of cognitive deterioration, opioid usage should be reduced or stopped. Because mental status is a universal precursor to respiratory depression it is unnecessary and unwise to wait for respirations to actually slow down. Alternative methods of pain control should be pursued.

ASSESSMENT

Opioid medications can reduce both the inspiratory drive and the quantity and quality of a patient's breathing. Thus, the health care provider should carefully **assess all facets of the respiratory process.** Count the patient's respiratory rate for one full minute (as opposed to shorter periods multiplied to obtain a per-minute rate) to capture any irregular variation and ensure accuracy. Observe the quality of respirations, which should be deep and regular, as opposed to shallow, episodically apneic, or otherwise of poor quality. Respirations should not fall below eight per minute. Assessment of the patient's level of consciousness (to detect subtle changes in sedation as well as any deterioration in mental status) should be repeated frequently (once every hour). If breathing has not slowed but changes in the patient's mental status have occurred, appropriate steps to revise the opioid therapy should take place. Alternative reasons for any change in mental status should also be considered and addressed as necessary.

MANAGEMENT

If a patient's respiratory rate has dropped below the standard rate of eight (8) respirations per minute, or where respirations have become shallow and of poor quality, or if the mental status of the patient is markedly abnormal, then **reversal of the opioid medication** is indicated. Naloxone should be administered. Naloxone is typically administered in small, frequent increments, although it can be administered quickly in cases of emergency. By titrating naloxone slowly, the nurse can reverse the respiratory side effects without entirely reversing the analgesia. When reversal takes place, the patient should continue to be monitored closely because the duration (i.e., half-life) of some opioids is longer than naloxone and the naloxone may need to be repeated. If rapid reversal takes place an increase in sympathetic drive, hypertension, tachycardia, rapid respirations, decreased gastrointestinal motility and hypercoagulability may occur. Alternative methods of analgesia should then be implemented.

NAUSEA

Nausea can be caused by many factors; thus, the specific cause of nausea should always be investigated. Any opioid administered via any route can cause nausea. With opioid administration, nausea tends to be present when patients are ambulatory rather than when they are recumbent. This may be due to the result of opioid-enhanced labyrinthine sensitivity to motion. Nausea should be assessed on a regular schedule with patients who are receiving opioid therapy. Individuals who suffer from very mild renal insufficiency may become nauseous with even small doses of morphine sulfate. Therefore, patients with even mild renal insufficiency should be monitored more closely for nausea.

MANAGEMENT

If nausea is reported the prescribed opioid may be changed. Various opioids produce different side effects and to differing degrees, so eliminating opioid therapy on the basis of nausea alone should be unnecessary. Also, antiemetics can be administered, when prescribed, although they may induce sedation. Antihistamines can also be administered, if ordered, though these too may augment sedation. If a patient is using a PCA device, decreasing their individual bolus dose or infusion rate may also help to decrease nausea. If nausea is severe, naloxone or nalbuphine (both opioid antagonists) can be administered slowly and in low doses to reverse the nausea without reversing the pain control. If nausea is related to ambulation, scheduling dosages of medication around periods of inactivity carefully may help reduce the incidence of nausea.

> **Review Video: Nausea and Vomiting**
> Visit mometrix.com/academy and enter code: 631968

URINARY RETENTION

Urinary retention commonly occurs with systemically administered opioids. The detrusor muscle at the floor of the bladder is relaxed by opioids, causing an inability to void. A physician or advanced practice nurse should evaluate the patient for possible mechanical urinary obstruction before the symptom is attributed to opioid therapy. Urinary retention is very uncomfortable for the patient and attempts at resolution should be made quickly.

Resolution is typically achieved by reducing the opioid dosage or changing the opioid all together. There are certain medications that induce contraction of the bladder (e.g., bethanechol chloride) which can be administered if they are prescribed. Bladder catheterization (usually done only once) relieves the problem, but because of its invasive nature it does expose the patient to the risk of developing a urinary tract infection.

PRURITUS

Pruritus is defined as severe itching. Pruritus can be attributed to hypersensitivity or allergy to the drug itself, or to the vehicle or medium through which the drug was delivered. However, only very rarely is a patient truly allergic or sensitive to opioid medication. Management of pruritus should begin by stopping the opioid administration. Dispensing antihistamine, as ordered, will typically increase sedation but will also help with the itching itself. Further, an opioid antagonist can be administered, per a physician's order. Slowly titrating the antagonist will decrease the side effect of itching while still maintaining analgesia. Because opioids are different and their side effects vary, changing to a different opioid with less likelihood to induce pruritus is prudent.

CONSTIPATION

Both pain and opioid treatment slow intestinal peristalsis, and immobility, poor diet and dehydration can also cause **constipation**, thus constipation is seen as one of the most common side effects of opioid therapy. To assess for constipation, a patient's bowel sounds should be routinely monitored as well as their elimination patterns (both baseline and during opioid therapy). Proper management of constipation secondary to opioid therapy and pain should utilize many modalities. Ensure that the patient is adequately hydrated and ambulates frequently, and is taking a high fiber diet, will help peristalsis to return to normal and relieve constipation. Stool softeners should be given routinely and peristaltic agents may be considered as well. Using an opioid antagonist to reverse the unwanted side effect of constipation can be effective and, if titrated slowly, the analgesic effects of the morphine can be retained.

SEDATION

Sedation is typically manifested as somnolence and mental clouding. It is a common side effect when opioid therapy is initiated and/or escalated. Co-analgesics such as antidepressants, anticonvulsants, benzodiazepines, antihistamines and phenothiazines may cause this problem to persist. The origin of any sedation should first be determined to rule out physiologic changes, central nervous system abnormalities, or metabolic instability. Where sedation is opioid induced, the opioid may be changed or the dosage altered provided adequate analgesia is maintained. If not, adjuvant medications should be added to a lower opioid dose. Psychostimulants may also be ordered (e.g., caffeine and dextroamphetamine, and methylphenidate) to offset the sedative side effects of opioid administration.

CONTACT DERMATITIS, MYOCLONUS, AND HYPERALGESIA

Contact dermatitis may occur when topical anesthetics such as benzocaine, dibucaine and lidocaine are used. These preparations are limited to use on the mucus membranes and skin. Contact dermatitis may occur with use of a patch-based preparation. A burning, itching or stinging with redness may be present at the site of application. The burning can be intense enough to discontinue therapy.

Myoclonus is defined as uncontrollable spasms of a particular muscle or muscle groups and can be seen at high doses of opioids.

Opioid-induced **hyperalgesia** is an excessive sensitivity to mildly noxious stimuli or an augmented response to previously non-painful stimuli. It is most common in patients receiving in long-term opioid therapy. At the end of life, the presence of one or both of these side effects may prohibit the use of opioids for pain control. Changing the opioid of choice, lowering the dosage and using co-analgesics and adjuvant medications may allow for resolution of the symptoms while maintaining analgesia.

Delirium

Delirium induced solely by opioid therapy is rare. Its cause is usually multifaceted. Delirium is typically linked with a rapidly changing mental status, and disorientation and agitation are common features. It is different than sedation, as the patient's mental status will fluctuate rather than stay constant or simply deteriorate and agitation, rather than somnolence, is prominent. Delirium also presents with the following signs and symptoms: acute onset, marked inattention, disordered thinking and speech, and an altered level of consciousness. Delirium is often mistakenly blamed on opioid therapy. In point of fact, many drugs prescribed for pain (tricyclic antidepressants and benzodiazepines) may be the cause. Further, underlying health changes (fever, infection, dehydration, etc.) may readily precipitate or worsen delirium. A thorough assessment should be completed before discontinuation of an opioid analgesic takes place. Neuroleptics can be used to treat the symptoms of delirium.

Side Effects of NSAIDs

Every patient should be screened for potential **toxicity to non-steroidal anti-inflammatory drugs.** NSAIDs can cause gastroduodenal irritation and ulceration, renal cortical ischemia, hepatotoxicity and platelet dysfunction.

Non-steroidal anti-inflammatory drugs administered for pain can cause the following: dyspepsia (imperfect or painful digestion), abdominal discomfort, heartburn, nausea, vomiting, loss of appetite, etc. Most of these symptoms can be managed effectively by prophylactically taking the medications with food. If this does not correct the problem, an oral antacid or other medication to counteract the indigestion should be prescribed. There is always a risk of ulceration with NSAID therapy. This risk increases with age, previous difficulty taking NSAID drugs, a history of peptic ulcer disease, and smoking.

NSAID treatments also interfere with platelet aggregation. This can cause excessive bruising and bleeding which can take place both internally and externally. Aspirin is the most dangerous NSAID when considering impaired platelet aggregation. Aspirin irreversibly damages the platelet, causing platelet impairment that lasts the lifetime of the platelet (four to seven days). By comparison, other NSAIDs usually cause a decrease in platelet aggregation for only two additional days after therapy has discontinued. Because NSAIDs can cause gastrointestinal ulceration and affect platelet aggregation, gastrointestinal bleeds are common side effects of NSAID therapy. Elderly patients are at particular risk.

Risk of Hepatotoxicity

It is not uncommon for a patient being treated with non-steroidal anti-inflammatory drugs (NSAIDs) to show **elevations in hepatic transaminase levels.** Patients suffering from juvenile rheumatoid arthritis or systemic lupus erythematosus are at a higher risk. These findings, however, are not considered clinically significant unless one of the following occurs: elevations of hepatic transaminase levels exceed two to three times the upper normal limit, serum albumin falls, or prothrombin times are altered. Patients at risk for liver toxicity should be monitored very carefully, as overt liver failure, although rare, has occurred with NSAID therapy. All patients should be evaluated within eight to twelve weeks after NSAID treatment begins, with further laboratory blood testing if symptoms or conditions warrant.

SIDE EFFECTS ON RENAL FUNCTION

Non-steroidal anti-inflammatory drugs can also have effect on the **kidneys**. Changes in the excretion of sodium, alteration of tubular function, potential interstitial nephritis, and reversible renal failure due to alterations in filtration rate and renal plasma flow can all occur with the use of NSAID therapy. All non-steroidal anti-inflammatory drugs have been proven to interfere with ongoing medical management of existing hypertension and heart failure. Increases in blood pressure are seen with all NSAIDs in patients with known hypertension, while patients with normal blood pressure incur no change. Because of the potential complications, the kidney function of all NSAID patients with renal complications should be routinely tested and monitored very carefully. Specific parameters should be set for creatinine levels and discontinuation of therapy in these patients.

> **Review Video: Renal Cancer**
> Visit mometrix.com/academy and enter code: 299089

CENTRAL NERVOUS SYSTEM SIDE EFFECTS

Non-steroidal anti-inflammatory drugs may cause side effects that impact the **central nervous system**. Aseptic meningitis, psychosis, sedation, confusion, headache, depression and cognitive dysfunction are included on that list. Elderly patients are at greater risk for such effects. Tinnitus, a ringing, hissing, roaring, buzzing or tinkling sound in the ear, is commonly reported. Again, this is more commonly found in the elderly patient. Some elderly and pediatric patients may report hearing loss as well. When tinnitus is reported, dosages of the prescribed NSAID should be decreased and this will usually alleviate the symptom. Monitor the patient for changes in mental status, level of consciousness, reports of tinnitus, mood changes or confusion and headaches.

POTENTIAL TO PERPETUATE ASTHMA AND POTENTIAL FOR ANAPHYLAXIS

Non-steroidal anti-inflammatory drugs (NSAIDs) work by inhibiting prostaglandin synthesis in local tissues. The exact mechanism of action is unclear, but asthma symptoms are known to increase. One theory postulates that COX-1 (cyclooxygenase) activity is inhibited by NSAID therapy this and is followed by a decrease in the synthesis of prostaglandins that contribute to bronchodilation.

NSAIDs may also function as "haptens" (immune-response triggers), capable of inducing **allergic sensitization** and anaphylaxis or anaphylactoid reactions, including those of a respiratory nature. Further, their COX-1 inhibition effects may secondarily induce other cross-reactions and side effects. Patients with allergic rhinitis, nasal polyposis, and/or a history of asthma are at particular risk of respiratory reactions.

Nonacetylated salicylates are regard as a safe choice for these patients, even though at high dosages these drugs may also inhibit prostaglandin synthesis enough to induce an anaphylactic reaction in highly sensitive patients.

Side Effects of Tricyclic Antidepressants

Tricyclic antidepressants block muscarinic, adrenergic and histamine receptors, leading to their more common side effects. **Anticholinergic symptoms** (i.e., dry mouth, constipation, blurred vision, and urinary retention) are common among this class of drug. Patients with narrow-angle glaucoma or benign prostatic hypertrophy should be treated carefully. Sedation and orthostatic hypotension (i.e., a drop in blood pressure upon standing) are also common side effects of these drugs. Elderly patients may be particularly at risk with these side effects. Appetite stimulation is also a side effect, and therefore weight gain may occur. Patients who suffer from postural hypotension, tachycardia, impotence, and priapism, gynecomastia in males, urinary retention, blurred vision, confusion, hallucinations and excessive sedation should discontinue treatment. Altered cardiac conduction with prolongation of the QT interval, tachycardia, ventricular arrhythmias and hypotension are relevant cardiovascular concerns. All patients over forty years of age should receive an electrocardiogram prior to treatment.

Side Effects of Acetaminophen

Acetaminophen is an easily accessible over-the-counter medication that is very safe. The incidence of adverse effects is less than 1% at a normal dose. The drug does, however, carry with it some potentially lethal side effects and drug interactions. The greatest risk is hepatic toxicity, which is even greater for those patients who regularly drink alcohol. A thorough history should be taken and honest alcohol intake should be ascertained before acetaminophen therapy is initiated. Dosages should be limited when alcohol intake is significant. Patients should be educated on dosing instructions because hepatic toxicity can also occur in patients who do not consume alcohol but have been exposed to large doses of acetaminophen. Acetaminophen may also mask infection because of its antipyretic affects.

Side Effects of Corticosteroids

Corticosteroids are effective in providing long term pain relief. They also cause many side effects including hyperglycemia, weight gain and neuropsychiatric side effects (such as dysphoria, euphoria and delirium). Myopathy (an abnormal condition of striated muscles) can also be a side effect with corticosteroid use. Osteoporosis is seen with long-term use and should be monitored carefully. Long term use can also result in immunosuppression, mood and behavior disturbances and fractures secondary to osteoporosis. Capsaicin is a topical preparation of corticosteroid but it can be prohibitive because of the intense burning sensation it causes on initial applications. Compliance, and therefore successful treatment, can become impeded by this unfortunate burning. Therefore, ongoing assessments should take care to ascertain compliance.

Side Effects of Anticonvulsant Medications

Anticonvulsants have few side effects and most that do occur are relatively benign. These drugs can, however, cause sedation and hypotension along with dizziness, ataxia (defective muscular coordination) and confusion. This usually occurs when escalation of the therapeutic dose has occurred too rapidly. Other side effects include headache and constipation, although these are less common. Because of these side effects these drugs are best administered at bed time during the initial dose titration process. While this drug does not cause renal impairment or decreased renal function, because of the drug's particular pharmacokinetics it is best to adjust the dose in patients suffering from renal failure. Patients should be evaluated for these side effects and titration of the dose slowed or discontinued, as/if needed.

Allergic Reactions

Management of **allergic reactions** begins before any drug has been administered. Ideally, a thorough history and physical would take place prior to any drug being prescribed. Information regarding allergies including drug allergies should be fully reviewed. Of course, in many medical emergencies obtaining a complete history and physical may not be realistic. In urgent situations, patients and family members should be questioned regarding allergies as well as looking for any medical alert bracelets or necklaces indicating such. Allergies should be noted on all files pertaining to the patient as well as being added to identifying markers on the patient during their admission (e.g., ID bracelets, etc.). Keep in mind that allergic reactions to medications take more than one exposure to the allergen before an allergic reaction would take place. Therefore, any drug given has the potential to create an allergic reaction.

Monitoring for the **signs and symptoms of an allergic reaction** should be done with every medication administered. Because there is no way to identify an unknown allergy until it occurs, and because sensitization (previous exposure) needs to take place prior to an allergic reaction being manifest, virtually every drug is a potential allergen. Symptoms of allergic reactions can range from rashes, hives, difficulty breathing, throat constriction, wheezing, coughing, sneezing and nasal congestion as well as full anaphylaxis. Diphenhydramine, epinephrine or corticosteroids should be readily available in case of systemic anaphylaxis in reaction to a drug administration. In most cases if an allergic reaction is suspected the administration of any questionable drugs should stop and a different course of therapy prescribed. A nurse has the responsibility to alert physicians to any possible allergic reactions.

Drug Interactions

Drug interactions are defined as a change in the amplitude or length of a response to one drug while another drug is present. As a result, there will be an increase or decrease in concentration of the drug at the site of action. There are many factors that cause drug interactions. When a change in the metabolism of a drug takes place, or the drug is displaced from plasma proteins, a drug interaction can occur. If there is poor gastrointestinal absorption of the drug or if the individual has a level of renal dysfunction causing the excretion of the drug to be altered, then a drug interaction can occur. Certain changes in electrolyte balances or bodily fluid pH levels can cause interactions. Alterations in the pace of protein synthesis can also bring about a drug interaction. Finally, changes in receptor channels or receptor blocking channels can cause changes that would advance drug interactions.

Variables That Affect Adverse Drug Reactions

Many factors contribute to **drug interactions**. The age of the patient is an important factor in how drugs are metabolized, absorbed and excreted, and at what rates and with what levels of toxicity. The complexity of these issues can easily lead to an adverse drug reaction. Individuals with genetic factors (e.g., with specific enzyme deficiencies) may have idiosyncratic difficulties with certain drugs, causing them to face an adverse drug reaction. Outside of the patient, a drug itself is also subject to causing an adverse drug reaction. Further, the route of administration, the exact product formulation, and the amount of time the patient undergoes drug therapy, are all variables in potential drug reactions. Finally, there are also drug-induced diseases that produce causative factors favoring adverse drug reactions.

Non-Pharmacologic Pain Management

TENS Device

A **transcutaneous electrical nerve stimulation (TENS) device**, or "TENS unit" as it is often called, uses electrical impulses to reduce pain. The impulses are conducted through pads that are attached to the skin. The electrical impulses pass through the skin via electrodes connected to the pads. It is thought that the sensory nerves carrying pain messages are interrupted by these impulses. The patient should feel only vibrations during a TENS treatment, with the therapist looking for a broader, deeper sense of vibration, not a stronger one. The patient should never feel pain from the TENS unit, as this will only reinforce the existing pain message. The TENS unit can be placed at the site of pain, or along the root of the nerve that innervates the painful area. There are no significant side-effects associated with the use of a TENS unit, and it can be used for both chronic and acute pain conditions. However, a TENS unit would not be helpful in treating poorly localized pain or psychogenic pain.

A transcutaneous electrical nerve stimulation (TENS) unit should not be used as the only method of treatment for moderate to severe pain. It should also not be used if a cardiac pacemaker has been fitted, or before the thirty-seventh week of pregnancy, unless otherwise directed by a physician. It should not be used over a metal prosthesis or if the patient is found to be allergic to conductive gel or electrodes. The pads for a TENS unit should not be placed on skin lesions, rashes or open wounds, or over carotid sinuses or on the throat. Do not use the TENS unit in the bath or shower or otherwise around water. The TENS unit is not designed for use while operating hazardous machinery or while driving. The patient must be cooperative and have the capacity to be educated on the safe use of the TENS unit for maximum effectiveness.

Superficial Hot and Cold Treatment Modalities

Superficial hot and cold treatment modalities are commonly used in the treatment of pain. Patients can independently use hot and cold treatments at home, which makes them versatile and widely recommended. Patients should only be encouraged to use these methods at home for indicated injuries. Generally, using cold (ice bags, ice massage) at the first sign of acute injury will help to decrease swelling when heat (water bottles, heating pads) later becomes the appropriate choice. Subsequent heat will cause an influx of chemicals that are advantageous to healing. Patients should be educated on how to look for possible burns on the skin and how to protect the skin from damage due to excessive heat and/or cold.

Physiological Effects of Heat

Heat therapy can be useful in the treatment of pain. It has physiological effects that are local, regional and distant. Locally, heat can increase the release of tissue inflammatory substances such as histamine, prostaglandin and bradykinin and thereby help relax vascular smooth muscles that aide in the process of vasodilation. Because of afferent thermoreceptor stimulation, sympathetic vascular tone is also more fully relaxed. When blood is warmed enough to reach the thermoregulatory mechanism in the hypothalamus, it causes an increase in metabolism and tissue recovery preparation. Tissue that is itself safely warmed will increase in elasticity and will decrease in viscosity. Thus, heat and applications of deep heat are included in this pain treatment modality.

Contraindications to Heat Treatment

If a patient is confused, disoriented, or vegetative, hot applications are contraindicated. If a patient is struggling with peripheral vascular disease, acute inflammation, tumors, an injury close to a growth plate, or if the skin is insensitive to temperature changes then heat preparations should be avoided. Patients with congestive heart failure should not be treated with immersion in a whirlpool.

Finally, it is important that the prospective patient for heat therapy can sense and express the perception of heat or the sensation of being burned. If a patient cannot perceive heat or burning because of cognitive compromise, inattention, or a peripheral nerve disorder they are at extremely high risk of burns and heat therapy should never be used.

METHODS OF EXTERNAL HEAT TREATMENT

There are several different **external heating devices** that can be employed to help decrease pain. Each method has different parameters for temperature variation and unique techniques for use. The following are three common heat therapy methods:

- **Hydrocollator hot packs** should 71 degrees Celsius (160 degrees Fahrenheit) and be wrapped in six to eight layers of toweling. Never lay a patient on the hot pack as the pressure of the body will prevent adequate dissipation of the heat. After five minutes the skin under the pack should be checked for excessive redness. If the skin is too red, extra toweling should be applied or the pack should be removed.
- **Paraffin dips** can be heated to 47 to 54 degrees Celsius. The patient can dip their extremities into the wax mixture eight to ten times, or have the mixture brushed on. Proper equipment should be used to prevent injury.
- **Water bottles** are easily self-limited for heat but should be sealed properly to prevent injury.

ULTRASOUND AS A MODE OF DEEP HEAT THERAPY

Repeated research has shown no clinical decrease of pain in patients who have used **ultrasound**. However, this treatment can affect tissue distensibility (flexibility), which may be advantageous. Ultrasound is generated when electrical current passes through crystals to cause vibrations and then sound waves. With different frequencies, ultrasound waves can penetrate 1-5cm into the tissue. As the ultrasound waves are passed through the tissue, they are absorbed or reflected depending on the makeup of the tissue. Different tissue temperatures will be reached, depending on the tissue's composition. Since ultrasound passes poorly through air, a gel must be used to improve conduction. The patient should perceive warmth during treatment, and treatment should be discontinued if the patient perceives a burning sensation.

STRETCHING AS A COMPONENT TO A PAIN THERAPY EXERCISE PROGRAM

The first step in an exercise program should be **stretching**. Flexibility should not be confused with strength or physical fitness. Flexibility is defined as the ability to move a joint smoothly throughout a full range of motion. With no inhibiting disease, muscles, tendons and the joint capsule are the only limiting factors in flexibility. However, injury, disease, neurological conditions (including hypertonicity), and excessive adipose tissue can limit flexibility. Stretching prevents soft tissue injury and should be the initial step in any exercise program. Stretching has been shown to decrease pain. Two types of stretch techniques should be employed:

- **Static stretch:** Slowly stretching the muscle to a point of discomfort and holding that position for sixty seconds. This technique is helpful the first few days following an injury.
- **Contract-and-relax stretch:** Maximum contraction of the muscle is maintained for ten seconds, followed by a slow stretch while contracting the opposing muscle group. This technique can be used with acute soft tissue injury.

Isometric, Isotonic, and Isokinetic Muscle Contractions

The following are categories of muscle contractions:

- **Isometric**: A muscle contraction in which the muscle develops significant tension but the muscle does not change its length. There are not as many daily implications for this type of muscle contraction.
- **Isotonic**: A muscular contraction where constant tension is maintained by the muscle group by changing its length during the action. All or part of the normal range of motion is utilized while lifting a constant amount of weight (e.g., bicep curl with a dumbbell). There are two types of isotonic contractions:
  - Concentric contraction – muscle shortening.
  - Eccentric contraction – muscle lengthening.
- **Isokinetic**: Where the muscle contracts and shortens at the same rate or speed under variable loads. Usually achieved through specialized equipment that senses movement and increases or decreases the load to maintain consistent speed. The goal is to increase strength more quickly, and to strengthen the muscle equally throughout the range of motion.

Strength Training in a Pain Therapy Exercise Program

Strength training can improve posture, increase range of motion, and reduce some kinds of pain. Many people are resistant to the idea of strength training. Lack of knowledge, fear of the unknown, or the misconception that they get adequate "exercise" in their daily lives contributes to this resistance. The research literature states clearly that every day activities of living will not produce adequate flexibility, strength, endurance or bone density. Organized, intense exercise efforts are needed. In the beginning of a strength building treatment program (two to three weeks) strengthening occurs because of neuromuscular integration. After that, it occurs because of muscle hypertrophy. Exercises should be repeated to the point of muscle fatigue to improve strength. Those seeking pain relief should use considerable caution. Strength exercises should not be performed by those suffering from a fracture. Those with significant hypertension should be continually monitored, as strengthening exercises cause an abrupt rise in blood pressure. If a patient suffers from acute or unstable cardiopulmonary disease strength training is contraindicated.

Endurance Training in a Therapy Plan Involving Exercise

Endurance exercises will increase aerobic capacity (i.e., maximum oxygen uptake). The number and size of mitochondria in muscle cells also increase through endurance training. Further, the individual will benefit from increased blood flow to the muscles because of increased capillary structures and greater efficiency of blood flow. The heart and vasculature benefit by an increased stroke volume, expanded blood volume, a decreased resting heart rate, and decreased resting blood pressure (both diastolic and systolic). Endurance exercise has been shown to increase endorphin levels, thereby decreasing perceived pain. Short, frequent bouts of endurance exercise have been shown to be equally as effective as long, sustained exercise. Patients who have suffered marked deconditioning will be better served by beginning with small, manageable amounts of endurance exercise. Be sure to have participants fully educated on the form, safety and goals for each exercise.

Massage for Pain

The neurological mechanisms by which **massage** works to decrease pain are currently unknown. However, massage is thought to interfere with pain transmission and perception at the peripheral level. It is deeply relaxing, and can communicate warmth and caring to patients, thereby further decreasing their pain.

Positioning and Movement as Appropriate Treatment Methods for Pain

Positioning of a patient is the deliberate placement of the body into postures that maintain or help to facilitate normal physiological function. When muscles become atrophied because of lack of use, especially when related to pain, using movement and positioning interventions can help refurbish the integrity of the muscles, ligaments, joints and bones as well as nerves that are used for movement and daily activities. Neurophysiologic reflexes are also activated by range of motion exercises, which may in turn reduce pain.

Spinal Cord Stimulator

The dorsal columns are responsible for relaying pain messages in the spinal cord. **Spinal cord stimulators** use electrical stimulation to interrupt these messages. A patient is first sedated and then an electrode is placed in the epidural space close to the dorsal column. The placement is then confirmed by X-ray. With placement confirmed, electrical impulses can now be used to change the pain messages that are relaying in the dorsal columns. It should be emphasized that this procedure is highly invasive and requires a commitment to long-term care and follow-up. Further, the instruments can incur site slippage and broken wires, and may precipitate infection at the placement site or elsewhere. Thus, patients should continue with concurrent treatment modalities and be carefully educated on how to use the stimulator. Spinal cord stimulators are most commonly used for patients with angina, peripheral vascular disease, Complex Regional Pain Syndromes (CRPS) and Failed Back Syndrome with radicular pain.

Range of Motion Exercises for Immobile Patients

Range-of-motion exercises stimulate mechanisms within the body that reduce pain. An individual who has been rendered immobile should receive daily range-of-motion exercises as a component of their pain treatment plan. These exercises should be conducted with all the joint groups, including a sustained stretch at the end of the range of motion (the end of a patient's range of motion should be considered where structural resistance is felt). These exercises should be conducted by trained personnel. Special consideration should be given to those patients who are afflicted with osteoporosis, as they are at high risk of fractures. Patients who are not entirely immobile may also benefit from active-assisted range-of-motion exercises in which the patient actively contributes to the stretching.

Cognitive-Behavioral Intervention

Cognitive-behavioral pain treatment is based upon several theoretical components. First, it assumes that patients are active participants and not passively reacting to their pain processes. Second, thoughts are believed to influence mood and have an effect on the physiologic process of the body. Third, it also assumes that patients should be active participants in changing their maladaptive thoughts (in this case, regarding their chronic pain). Indeed, cognitive-behavioral treatment hinges on the belief that individuals are able to learn more advantageous ways of thinking, feeling and behaving in response to those feelings and thoughts. Cognitive-behavioral therapy generally takes place in a formal individual or group therapy setting, on either an inpatient or outpatient basis. Again, the goal is to help the patient change maladaptive thoughts regarding their pain and their subsequent pain-related functioning.

The **first step** in cognitive-behavioral therapy is known as **the psycho-educational phase.** It is here that the care-givers enlist the patient as an active participant in the process of their own recovery and rehabilitation. The mind-body model of pain is introduced, including the stress-reactivity and the pain-stress cycles, to help the patient identify which thoughts, attitudes and beliefs may be contributing to their suffering and making their pain more difficult to manage. Negative thoughts and beliefs regarding their pain can significantly inhibit a patient's belief that they can become well. Examining and identifying such thoughts is imperative to challenging them, in the ultimate hope of teaching oneself new and more advantageous thoughts, beliefs, and behavior patterns.

The **second** or **skills-building phase** of cognitive-behavioral therapy involves developing cognitive strategies to better recognize those negative thoughts and beliefs that can impact on their recovery and healing. Next, these negative thoughts are replaced with positive self-affirming ones ("I can handle this," or "Things aren't exactly how I'd like, but I can still do many things," etc.) Training one's mind to think positively regarding one's unique pain processes will serve to encourage treatment on all fronts.

Coping strategies may also be taught during the skills-building phase. Relaxation, stress management, anger management, assertiveness training and pacing are all good options, especially when a patient must confront regular (pain stimulated) catalysts to negative thoughts that increase autonomic arousal, musculoskeletal tension, and thereby escalate the patient's pain experience.

Cognitive-behavioral therapy enters its **third phase** (the **application phase**) when cognitive skills, behavioral techniques and coping strategies are combined and decisively applied in battling thoughts, beliefs and behaviors with negative outcomes for chronic pain management. Learning these skills will hopefully help the patient to become more adaptive as their pain processes continue and change. At this juncture, patients can use the tools and techniques they have acquired as a blue print in gauging their thoughts, beliefs and behaviors and the consequent impact on their pain. Cognitive-behavioral therapy should not be viewed as a cure for chronic pain, but rather as a tool for dealing with the constant or erratic intrusion of the pain process.

Spiritual Care

Patients come to health care providers with a wide variety of **spiritual beliefs and needs.** While it is not appropriate to judge, change, or thwart their spiritual needs, it is important to support their spiritual needs in relation to the healing process. Thus, it is important to emphasize and value the patient's beliefs, particularly where this may encourage them to take an active part in their healing, rehabilitation and recovery process. Special considerations should be made for spiritual practices (hours of prayer or clothing considerations, etc.) that are reasonable and do not cause harm. Supporting a patient and their family in their spiritual needs can help the patient to continue moving forward in the healing process.

Relaxation Techniques

Relaxation techniques have long been related to success in the treatment of chronic pain. Relaxation can help decrease muscle tension that may be contributing to pain. Muscle tension-relaxation exercises, passive muscle relaxation, deep breathing exercises, autogenic exercises, imagery and visualization are all used for chronic pain management. Three particular strategies include:

- **Visual imagery:** The patient is encouraged to visualize a place or activity. They are encouraged to use all their senses: smell the air, taste the food, hear the noises, see the surroundings associated with their unique place or activity.
- **Autogenic exercises:** The patient uses a repetitive mantra ("I feel light" or "heavy" or "warm", etc.) to tune into the body, coupled with positive affirmations and imagery. It is intended to induce relaxation and healing.

- **Breathing techniques:** In through the nose and out through the mouth, being sure to breathe in as much as one breathes out. These exercises allow the patient to be distracted and to self-soothe when the need arises.

Acupuncture

Acupuncture is based on the theory that there are patterns of energy that flow through the body that necessary for maintaining health. Disruptions of these patterns, per acupuncture theory, results in disease. Acupuncture is thought to correct these imbalances using the placement of needles in the "meridian system" of acupuncture points. There is an accumulation of research that supports acupuncture. Much of it is as strong as the research supporting Occidental medicinal therapies. However, acupuncture also carries a lower incidence of ill effects than many pharmacological counterparts. Acupuncture is widely supported for patients suffering from fibromyalgia, headache, menstrual cramps, myofascial pain, osteoarthritis, low back pain, carpal tunnel syndrome and epicondylitis. Patients should look for someone who has been properly trained and credentialed by a state agency.

Environmental Factors in the Healing Process

Florence Nightingale developed her concept of nursing around revising and enhancing the **environment** of her patients to suit their needs. For Nightingale the environment consisted of ventilation, light, clean water, warmth, noise control and management of fluids and odors. While certainly some of these environmental concerns have come a long way and are no longer considered primary risk factors, others are still at issue and can play a significant role in the reduction of discomfort in the pain patient. Adjusting lighting, noise and temperature should still take place to suit each individual patient in today's world, as well as improving comfort with positioning, pillows and assistive devices. Listening to patients and giving them choices regarding their environment, especially while they are under the stress of pain and illness, may well begin the process of comfort.

Homeopathy

The basis of **homeopathy** is the belief that a symptom is a positive sign that the body is actively fighting a disease process. Thus, homeopathic treatment is designed to encourage symptoms that are occurring, thereby helping the body thwart the disease process. It is also believed that each body is unique, as are the symptoms, which thus require a uniquely prescribed remedy. This fact makes studying homeopathy challenging at best. While there is some evidence that homeopathic methods are effective for some conditions (i.e., with asthma, allergy and infantile diarrhea), but its effectiveness in pain relief is not well defined.

Magnetotherapy and Chiropractic Therapy

Magnetotherapy is the process of applying magnets or using magnetism in treating symptoms of disease. While some studies have claimed effective results, others have found no benefit or have ascribed any apparent benefits to a placebo effect. To date, there is no consensus that there is any medical benefit to this therapy, although some mainstream medical practitioners do continue to prescribe such treatments.

Chiropractic medicine is a theory of health care that is focused on the belief that the structure and function of the body are symbiotic. When the structure of the body is not aligned properly, or positioned optimally then the function of the body will decrease and the individual will experience maladaptive symptoms. The spinal column and the nervous system have a significant relationship, since nerve energy is expressed and transmitted through these tissues. Chiropractic medicine seeks to improve overall health through the restoration and maintenance of the structure of the body.

Some chiropractic approaches do appear to relieve pain, although many modalities and claims remain unproven.

THERAPEUTIC TOUCH

Therapeutic touch (TT) is based on the theory that our bodies are surrounded by an energy field. TT is considered a nursing technique that manipulates the human energy field through touch to settle imbalances. There are three steps included in the therapeutic touch process:

1. The nurse calmly brings him or herself to mental and emotional center, a place where he or she wishes to be of service and is compassionate.
2. The nurse will then assess the patient's energy field with his or her own hands (yet this is a non-contact process). Abnormal areas in the energy field are detected by energy feel.
3. The nurse will then use therapeutic touch, a non-contact process of manipulating the energy field over the affected area.

Research published in the Journal of the American Medical Association (Rosa L, Rosa E, Sarner L, Barrett S. A Close Look at Therapeutic Touch. JAMA;1998; 279:1005-1010) concluded this therapeutic modality to be inefficacious.

Important Terms

Palliative Sedation—Administered for the purpose of alleviating or eliminating pain and stress without curing the underlying precipitating factors. In the case of palliative care, sedation may be particularly desirable to calm the patient and reduce their anxiety.

Moderate Sedation—A drug induced state in which the patient's level of consciousness is diminished. They remain able to respond to voice commands with little physical stimulation, and there is no need for ventilation or concern for circulation and heart function.

General Anesthesia—A drug induced state in which the patient has a loss of consciousness and is not responsive or arousable even by painful stimulation. A patent airway will be needed as the patient cannot spontaneously respire on their own. Cardiovascular function may also be impaired.

Side Effect—A dose-related predictable reaction to a medication. These effects have been frequently observed in individuals who have taken the medication. Side effects that are expected are based upon the pharmacologic activity of the drug in the body.

Adverse Effect—The development of an undesired side effect or toxicity caused by the administration of certain drugs. Adverse effects can occur suddenly or they may take days to develop. Adverse reactions, drug interactions and drug reactions all refer to adverse drug effects.

Allergic Reaction—A hypersensitivity reaction to a medication that has been administered. It is an acquired, abnormal immune response to a medication. Allergic reactions take more than one exposure to the allergen (medication) for the allergic reaction to ensue.

Additive Effect—The sum effect when two drugs with similar pharmacokinetics are taken.

Synergistic Effect—The combined effect of two drugs which, when acting alone, do not create the same effect as when taken together. An increased effect is created by administering the two drugs together.

Potentiation—When one drug increases the result of a second drug. One drug is taken to enhance the effect of a different drug.

Toxic Effect—Extreme drug levels occurring when a patient takes or is administered too much of a medication.

Competitive Antagonism—A drug with the same attraction for the identified receptor as the agonist (i.e., opioids and naloxone). Competition for the receptor site reduces the effect of the agonist (opioid) at the receptor site.

CONVERSIONS FOR MEASUREMENTS

The following are important conversions for nurses to know when calculating drug dosages:

- 1 kg = 2.2 lb
- 1 tsp = 5 mL = 60 gtts
- 1 mL = 1 cc
- 1000 mL = 1L
- 1 tbsp = 3 tsp = 15 mL
- 1 oz = 30 mL = 2 tbsp
- 1 cup = 15 fluid oz

Professional Practice

Patient, Caregiver, and Family Education

PATIENT EDUCATION

Patient education is defined as the facilitation of voluntary changes in behavior that are favorable to the patient's health and wellness by a combination of learning experiences.

Goals and objectives of patient education should include the improvement of pain relief and an increased knowledge and awareness of their pain and methods to manage it. Patient education should serve to dispel myths and misconceptions including those regarding pain control and medicinal drug use, among others. Patients receiving education regarding their pain treatment plans should become more compliant and adhere to the plan more successfully. Patient education can also serve to help patients develop pain control techniques that they can utilize themselves. Patient education should include the family and focus on the patient and their role in the family.

NEEDS ASSESSMENT PRIOR TO PATIENT AND FAMILY EDUCATION

A **needs assessment** should be completed before any patient teaching or family education is attempted. A patient's physical condition will have a significant impact on their ability to focus and learn. Prior knowledge of the disease and therapy should be ascertained, as well as the accuracy of the information. A patient's access to health care and level of social support should also be evaluated. A patient's demographics should be taken into consideration, including the patient's family status, employment history (past and present) and their formal education. A pediatric patient will have different needs than a middle-aged man or an elderly woman, and stages of development should be evaluated. Everyone has different preferences regarding information and education and educators should note these specifics. The patient's emotional response to their disease process or injury will impact their ability to learn, as will their cultural beliefs, the meaning of pain, and any spiritual beliefs they harbor.

SPECIAL CONSIDERATIONS

Children have different maturity levels and the information and educational presentation should be adapted to meet their needs. They may also have special needs in regards to cognitive development, language development, reading ability, motor function and concrete thinking. Their learning abilities will also differ, and consideration for the way they learn best should be included.

Adolescents also have different maturity levels for similar chronological ages. Their abilities to think abstractly and their reading levels may differ as well. As with all populations, adolescents will have learning preferences and these should be accommodated within other age-appropriate parameters.

Elderly patients experience cognitive, sensory and psychomotor changes as they age. Their information-integration and response time may be longer and they should be given adequate time to respond. Also, their energy level and potential for fatigue should be constantly evaluated. Patients will have difficulty learning when they are low on energy and/or are fatigued.

TYPES OF LEARNERS

While there are three **types of learners** (auditory, visual and kinesthetic) there is additional information to keep in mind regarding what and how much most people remember when they are exposed to information. People tend to remember only 10% of what they read. They remember 20% of what they hear and 30% of what they read and hear. Individuals will remember 50% of what they hear and see and 70% of what they say or repeat back in some way. Up to 90% of what they say and do will be remembered. Obviously, these numbers will differ according to the individual, but generally, the more ways that a person is exposed to information, the better chance he or she has of retaining it.

Auditory Learners

Auditory learners are one of three types of learners. They learn best when listening to a lecture or a fast-paced exchange of information between people. These learners prefer group discussion, particularly where many other points of view are presented and discussed. Often in group discussions stories and/or jokes are told that reiterate the information presented. Auditory learners will rely on these anecdotes to help them retain the information. They may also rely on verbal cues or mnemonic devices for remembering information. Presenting an auditory learner with videos, books, diagrams or other visual information will not aid their learning nearly as much as conversations, discussions, lectures and stories.

Visual Learners

There are several different methods in which information is processed, and there are at least three different types of learners. **Visual learners** are one type. Visual learners learn best when they are presented with information in the form of graphs or other illustrated information such as maps, written material, diagrams or videos. They like being close to the presenter (often sitting in the front row of seats) so they can see and interpret the facilitator's gestures and facial expressions. These cues add to their learning process. They are comfortable taking notes and will often ask for repetition of verbal instructions. The verbal instructions are harder for them to process; thus, it does take repeating.

Kinesthetic Learners

Kinesthetic learners are one of three types of learners. They learn best by moving and manipulating items and trying tasks. They prefer to "just do it," versus having a discussion or watching a video. These learners do better with frequent breaks in the presentation of information and may shake a leg, rock in their seat, stand at the back of the room or find other ways to move about when being presented with information in a lecture format. These learners do best with hands on experience and need physicality in a topic for optimum learning. These learners also make hand gestures often and prefer role play as a method of learning over discussion groups or information presented in diagrams, graphs or videos.

Combining Learning Styles as Information Is Presented

While most people are believed to have a preference of one type of learning over another, there are people who learn best with a **combination** of all three types (auditory, visual and kinesthetic approaches). Ideally, a patient's learning preference would be assessed before any information was presented. In some health care situations this type of evaluative approach will fit easily into the setting and tasks at hand. However, in a hospital or acute care setting there is often no time to assess a patient's learning type. Also, when presenting information to a patient's family as well as to the patient themselves, there will most certainly be several learning styles present. Presenting information using all three methods (via books, diagrams, videos, lectures, hands on demonstrations, personal conversations, etc.) will serve best in situations where time is limited or when more than one person will be learning the information.

Tools to Help Retain, Compare, Visualize, and Reinforce Learning

Giving patients tools that can help them retain, analyze, visualize and reinforce information will help in the learning, decision making and implementation process. Using printed materials such as pamphlets, articles, pictures or posters will also be helpful. Employing adjunct videotapes, audiotapes and computer-assisted programs can help further augment the learning done in other settings and modalities (possibly lecture, discussion groups or demonstrations). Again, presenting information in a variety of ways will help accommodate all types of learners. Preparing checklists for patients to navigate their learning process will also be beneficial. Using articulated models, particularly for health education, can be very valuable. The human body is a complex and easily misunderstood organism, and using a model to help describe disease processes, pain syndromes and treatment modalities can help provide correct information and more readily dispel myths and misconceptions.

Concepts Regarding Adult Learning

Andragogy is the art and science of teaching adults. **Teaching adults** is different than teaching children in many ways, as adults are typically more facile in their learning processes. Adults are also self-directed, and they have a deeper history and a fund of experience and information that they bring to the learning process. This will affect their perception of the information presented and how they integrate that information into their own knowledge base. They often have a readiness to learn tasks that are specific to their social or familial role. They are usually seeking information to use for immediate application. This can be helpful when new medical skills are presented that they may need to learn. Adult learning begins with a subject-focus and moves toward a problem-solving focus with the addition of more information. With adults, a teacher is more of a facilitator, creating a climate conducive to learning, planning the learning process, and structuring the learning experience.

Health Belief Model and Transtheoretical Theory of Learning and Motivation

The **health belief model** of learning and motivation contends that an individual's actions toward health and wellness are dependent upon their beliefs. The impacting beliefs are as follows:

- Belief regarding a person's susceptibility or vulnerability to the ill-health condition, which lies at the origin of the problem.
- Belief regarding the severity of this problem and the potential impact on the individual's life.
- Belief that the benefit to acting on positive health behaviors is greater than the barriers to those positive behaviors.
- A confidence that the individual can perform the advantageous action.

There are prudent motivational stages and intentional changes requiring progression through these stages over a course of time. Thus, different stages will require active use of different agents of change. Modifications of cognition, affect, and behaviors will occasionally be necessary.

Principles of Motivation on Education

Motivation affects education directly in that information can be presented in a way that is conducive to an individual's unique learning needs and style and learning can be inhibited or even prohibited by lack or inadequate motivation on the part of the learner. Use these principles to help facilitate motivation in learners. Structure the information to enhance motivation. Provide the learner with profound reasons why the learning needs to take place, using imperative information first. Remember that with learning comes an expected level of anxiety. Mild anxiety is motivating, while severe anxiety is incapacitating and will prohibit learning. Assess for anxiety and plan learning around the findings. Encouraging the client to set realistic goals will help sustain their motivation; small successes are wonderful motivators! Both affiliation and approval are strong motivators.

IMPLEMENTATION OF INSTRUCTIONAL METHODS

Patients will respond to information in different ways depending on their unique style of learning. Many different **methods** can and should be used in an effort to maximize the transfer of information. Self-directed learning modules, such as videos on injury/pain specific exercises, can be used. These modules are presented to the patient individually, and they may work at their own pace to complete the information. There is no educational facilitator present. More formally, group discussion or didactic formats can be used, such as a group exercise session to teach injury/pain specific exercises. These groups would be led by the educator. Yet another method would be individual (one-on-one) teaching. Demonstrating the stretching and/or exercises and having the patient demonstrate them back can also hasten the learning process.

IMPLEMENTATION OF ACTIVITIES

Many people have an innate preference for how they like information to be presented for optimal learning. Using many different methods and **activities** when teaching can help reach all three types of learners (visual, auditory, and kinesthetic). Lectures in traditional formalized education settings are very helpful to some individuals. Those who enjoy the verbal presentation of information are typically auditory learners. Demonstrations, such as how to prepare medications for administration, can easily be added to the traditional lecture format, catching the eye of those who learn visually. Role play or a return to demonstrations will help the kinesthetic learner better assimilate information.

ROLE OF PATIENT EDUCATION IN MULTIDISCIPLINARY PAIN CENTERS

Multidisciplinary pain centers provide patient and family education as a core part of their therapeutic treatment plan. The primary educational goal is helping patients move from a place of helplessness or hopelessness regarding their pain to a place of greater control and comfort. Educational topics include:

- **Medications** including side effects, drug action, drug interactions and common myths and misconceptions.
- **Depression** and its link to chronic pain.
- **Body mechanics** and their preventative role in pain.
- **Coping strategies** from imagery, to relaxation exercises.
- **Stress management** and how to deal with anger and other difficult emotions.
- **Psychological factors** and how they impact the pain experience.

These and other topics of discussion and education are addressed at many multidisciplinary pain centers. Information is also focused on encouraging the patient to take an active role in their healing process and in making decisions for themselves in order to escape the victim role.

GUIDELINES FOR CANCER PAIN EDUCATORS

When educating cancer pain patients there are certain specific **guidelines** that should be followed. First, assure the patients that their pain can in fact, be relieved. Affirm also that pain control should be a therapeutic goal. Determining and discussing an individual's definition and/or meaning of pain in their life is important in helping to construct factual information around that definition. Many people are concerned about analgesic pain medication use, particularly opioid therapy, and myths and misconceptions regarding medicinal therapies, addiction and tolerance should be dispelled.

Teach patients how to effectively measure and report their pain to their health care providers, and give them information and expectations regarding effective communication of that pain.

Educating cancer patients on their pain will be challenging and may include many roadblocks. Cancer patients often expect and accept pain as a part of their disease process. This can make them more resistant to new and accurate information. Following the prescribed guidelines can make the task of educating cancer patients easier. Providing specific instructions on the administration, side effects and expected outcomes of each medication they are prescribed for pain is imperative. Instruction about potential adverse reactions and possible side effects should also come with information regarding the management of these ill effects, and the individual's role in that process. Educating cancer patients on the use of noninvasive treatment modalities is particularly helpful. It is an important way for that individual to gain back some control over their pain, and to secure additional tools to cope with their situation. Finally, emphasize that the goal of cancer pain treatment is not just pain relief but also pain prevention.

LIMITATIONS OF EDUCATION IN PAIN MANAGEMENT

There are many **limits in pain management education**. A patient being given knowledge and information does not mean he or she will put the information into practice. Further, individuals will often respond to an instructor in ways that are socially acceptable even if they disagree with the information they have been taught. In addition, an individual's disease process can have a significant impact on their learning. Learning may be particularly hampered if the prescribed treatments for healing and/or pain management are ineffective or if the patient is being under-treated. When these factors are in play it may become more difficult for the patient to accept or understand information and ultimately put that information into practice.

BARRIERS TO EDUCATION OF THE PATIENT AND FAMILY
ON THE PART OF THE HEALTH CARE PROVIDER

Many factors can influence the amount of teaching that can be successfully done with a patient and their family. Some of those factors include the **health care professional** and their role as educator. If pain management is not a priority for the provider, and if there is no specific accountability process, then adequate pain control goals may not be met. Health care providers are very busy and held to a tight time schedule. Thus, time constraints can also lead to barriers in educating patients. Misconceptions regarding pain, health care and education, as well as varying concerns and beliefs of the patient, family and staff will also have an impact on educating the patient and their family. Quality education requires a different skill set and knowledge base than other nursing duties. Not having the skills or knowledge required to be a successful educator will hinder the teaching and learning process.

ARISING FROM THE PATIENT

There are many factors that influence the teaching/learning process. A patient's age, sex, socioeconomic status and educational level will all have an impact on learning. A patient's culture can greatly impact their ability to learn, as can how the information is presented and who is present during teaching. Language barriers create significant difficulty in transferring information, and a patient's native language should be used in the teaching process whenever possible. Patients in pain often experience many burdensome emotions. Anxiety, grief and anger are all commonplace and can greatly impact the learning process. These emotions should be assessed for and accommodated when possible, as teaching should take place when they are at their lowest levels.

Some patients may be unreceptive to learning because their pain in some way provides them with a secondary gain (i.e., if it has come to serve a purpose in their life and they are reluctant to relinquish it). Patients who have experienced chronic pain also very often operate from an internal locus of control. They are trying to control their pain and experiences from inside themselves, sometimes making new information difficult to integrate. Finally, the environment can have significant impact on the learning process. Noise, temperature, timing, light and the distractions of visitors or activities in the room may all inhibit quality learning.

Many factors influence the process of education, and patients bring many of those factors to the table themselves. Patients who are suffering from mental illness, impaired cognitive function or personality disorders present unique difficulties for the health care provider. These challenges should be assessed for prior to education taking place and realistic learning goals should be set. Myths and misconceptions of the pain process, such as the misperceived nobility of pain, or the over acceptance of pain as an inevitable part of the disease process, and/or as a natural part of aging, etc., should all be assessed. If a patient has these or other equally maladaptive beliefs, the education process should start there. Patients may also hold negative beliefs about the use of analgesics (opioids in particular) that could affect their compliance. Provide patients with factual information regarding adverse outcomes, dependence, tolerance and addiction to assuage their fears about receiving analgesic treatment.

LITERACY AS A BARRIER TO PATIENT AND FAMILY EDUCATION

Literacy is easily taken for granted. Assessing a person's ability to read is a task that carries great emotional weight. Before beginning any educational program, calculate the patient's reading level using readability formulas and adapt information accordingly. For those patients at a low (or no) level of literacy use pictures, charts and diagrams as well as videos, and return often to demonstrations of specific skills. The amount of information should be limited to digestible bits of information for the patient's unique literacy level. Avoid using unnecessary medical terminology. What medical terminology needs to be used should always be followed with a complete explanation. Reinforce all teaching with examples, and avoid using idioms in teaching patients with literacy challenges. Whenever possible use direct positive statements, as well.

INTRACTABLE PAIN AND REFRACTORY SYMPTOMS

Intractable pain is defined as pain that is incurable or resistant to therapy. It is often associated with terminal disease processes and related pain at the end-of-life. Refractory symptoms associated with intractable pain near the end of life may include pain, dyspnea, nausea and vomiting. Patients may also experience refractory psychological symptoms (i.e., delirium), and they may experience both the physical and psychological symptoms. Many of these patients are suffering from pain that is not susceptible to treatment (i.e., the treatments do not provide adequate relief, they cannot provide relief within an allowable time frame, or they are associated with excessive or intolerable acute or chronic morbidity).

NEED FOR SEDATION AND OTHER PHYSICAL SYMPTOMS AT THE END-OF-LIFE

Sedation is the recommended treatment for intractable pain and the concurrent refractory symptoms near the end-of-life. Other related intractable pain relief treatments and terms include: pharmacologic hypnosis, morphine intoxication, and terminal sedation. Sedation is indicated when current treatments are unable to provide adequate relief, or the treatments themselves are associated with excessive or intolerable acute or chronic morbidity, or they are not expected to provide adequate pain relief within an allowable time frame. The intent of sedation is to provide relief from suffering in end-of-life care. Involving the patient (if possible), family and team of health care providers is important during the process of making decisions regarding using sedation as treatment for intractable pain. Opioids, benzodiazepines, barbiturates, neuroleptic drugs or combinations of these medications can be used to induce profound sedation (and thus pain relief) in these patients.

Important Education Concepts

IMPORTANCE OF ADEQUATE PAIN RELIEF AND POSSIBLE IMPEDING FACTORS

Inadequate pain relief is a phenomenon that has been well documented in many settings and circumstances, both in the past and the present. In the largest study ever completed on end-of-life care in the United States, known as the SUPPORT study, it was reported that 50% of conscious patients who died in a hospital experienced moderate to severe pain at least half of the time during their last three days of life. Even when a nurse was diligent in acknowledging pain and suggesting treatments for that pain, the pain typically remained untreated or under-treated. With pain treatment protocols becoming more prominent and with a renewed focus by the Joint Commission on pain relief, it appears evident that pain relief will continue to be a major issue. One major reason for inadequate pain relief is fear on the part of health care providers (both nurses and physicians) that they may be accused of causing a patient's death. Continuing education is needed to allay these fears and thereby improve pain management at and near the end of life.

PRINCIPLE OF DOUBLE EFFECT

Medications powerful enough to relieve great suffering are also powerful enough to compromise vital functions. Opioids administered at doses high enough to relieve profound suffering may compromise a patient's respiratory rate, blood pressure, temperature, metabolism (including healing and immune-response systems), and/or heart rate. When an action produces a desired primary "benefit" (pain relief) even while inducing unwanted secondary effects (compromised vital functions), it is referred to as a "double effect" scenario. The ethical **"Principle of Double Effect"** indicates that when an action is taken with the sole intent to provide an overwhelmingly necessary benefit, the unwanted secondary effects do not compromise the ethical integrity of the primary action. Administering medications with the sole intent to relieve suffering may have the unintended "double effect" of hastening death. However, in keeping with the Principle of Double Effect, this practice is not considered physician-assisted suicide nor euthanasia, and is permitted by law in the United States. Regardless of the stage of life, individuals have the right to relief of their pain.

The **four conditions** necessary to sustain the principle of double effects are:

1. The act must be morally good (or at least morally neutral). Regarding pain, the medication must be given with the sole intent to relieve intolerable suffering.
2. The good effect rather than the bad effect must be intended. Whereas the bad effect may be foreseen, it must not be intended. Thus, while pain medication may hasten death, the relief of intolerable pain must be the intent of the drug administration.
3. The bad effect must not be the means to the good effect (i.e., death must not be the direct means for the pain relief). Thus, only pain-relief medications would be acceptable, as opposed to intentionally poisonous medicines.
4. The good effect must outweigh the bad effect. When giving pain medications at the end-of-life, the outcome of relieving horrible and intolerable pain must outweigh the burden of a potentially hastened death, often most clear when death is already certain and imminent regardless of any action being taken.

DOUBLE EFFECT AND PHYSICIAN-ASSISTED SUICIDE

Many difficulties lie within the framework of the principle of double effect and its counterpart, **physician-assisted suicide**. One main criticism of the principle of double effect is the inability to confirm a health care provider's intent. One can claim intent to provide pain relief, when in fact the true intent is to hasten death (i.e., to provide physician-assisted suicide). Another challenge to the principle of double effect is the implicit assumption that some suffering that is worse than death. Not everyone subscribes to this belief, and it makes end-of-life palliative care legally, morally, and practically difficult. The United States Supreme Court has ruled that physician-assisted suicide is not a constitutional right, thus implicitly allowing the issue to be determined by individual states. Currently, eight states (California, Colorado, Hawaii, Montana, New Jersey, Oregon, Vermont, Washington) and the District of Columbia allow for some form of physician-assisted suicide.

Evaluation of Education

EVALUATION OF INFORMATION AND LEARNING

The process of teaching patients and their families is constantly evolving, with ever changing needs and goals. As **evaluation** takes place, new or amended goals can be developed. Asking specific questions regarding identified goals is one way to ascertain patient knowledge and information retention. For example, "Can you tell me three things that may aggravate your migraine headaches?" or "Can you tell me what you're going to do if your pain level goes higher than a "5" on our scale?" The nurse may also ask for a return demonstration on a skill that was taught. For example, "Can you show me how to do the relaxation breathing we worked on yesterday?" or "Can you teach me how to draw this medication up?" Having the patient "return the teaching" is a wonderful way to evaluate and reinforce their learning of the information previously given them.

EVALUATING PATIENTS

Evaluating the teaching process begins well before the information has ever been presented. For adequate evaluation to be accomplished, goals and priority outcomes must be set in advance. These goals should be established by the health care provider, with regard to the key learnings needed for ultimate success, and in consideration of the patient's age, socioeconomic level, formal education, cognitive ability and other deterministic learning and educational factors. The patient and their family should be made aware of these goals, and be allowed input into how and when the goals should be reached. The goals should be attainable and realistic in order to provide for success in patient teaching. As the patient's knowledge base improves and their confidence grows, new goals can be set for increased levels learning.

FINANCIAL CONCERNS

Many factors influence compliance and willingness to participate in pain treatment programs. **Financial concerns** are among the most common reasons why patients and their families delay or avoid health care. Inability to pay for medications, along with co-pays for tests, procedures, surgeries, or counseling may prove extremely prohibitive to successful pain treatment. Helping a patient and their family financially plan and prepare for their treatments is important to achieving success in pain management. Using a multidisciplinary approach will be most effective. Educate patients regarding low cost health care programs and subsidized medications, and encourage them to understand their health care rights and insurance policies. Pain is a multifaceted process. Stresses from finances, depression, sleep disturbances, etc., all will affect the success of pain control.

DIFFERENCES IN LEARNING AND INFORMATION EVALUATION FOR THE ELDERLY

Teaching the elderly holds unique challenges for the nurse. Aging affects individuals in many ways. Declines in the rate of information uptake, processing, and expression require the allotment of additional time in the educational process, and many elderly people are also affected by a decrease in visual acuity and hearing loss. Therefore, when engaging the learning process, elderly patients should be given ample time to answer questions, and educators should know that a lag in response time does not necessarily infer lack of understanding or competency. When evaluating competency for specific tasks it is important to ascertain if the task can realistically and safely be performed by an older patient. Muscle mass decreases, tremors, and loss of fine motor skills may render some skills impossible despite adequate academic learning and comprehension.

VARIATIONS IN EVALUATING LEARNING WITH CHILDREN

Teaching pediatric patients holds many unique challenges. Developmental stages will impact learning in much the same way that learning styles will. Information will need to be presented in a cognitively appropriate manner. To evaluate the pediatric client, developmental stage and cognitive ability will need to be carefully incorporated. Some tasks will be impossible for children to master because they may lack sufficient fine motor skill development. Realistic goals should be set at the outset of teaching. Further, parents and caregivers must also assume responsibility for the information to be learned by the child, in addition to learning the information themselves. Thus, evaluating the family's understanding and mastery of the information provided will also be important to overall successful outcomes.

CULTURAL CONSIDERATIONS WHEN EVALUATING LEARNING

Cultural considerations should be addressed at every level of nursing care. Every patient and his or her family will hold specific and unique beliefs regarding pain, its cause and acceptable resources for treatment. These beliefs will affect how they interpret, perceive and respond to injury and illness, as well as to the information and education given to them regarding their injury or illness. Assessing and understanding a patient's individual cultural needs will help to more meaningfully evaluate understanding, as well as ensuring that any proposed plan of action and/or education is culturally appropriate and acceptable. For example, many cultures hold strict definitions of gender roles. Women are the caretakers and men make the decisions for the family. In such cultures, women may be hesitant to gather information and make decisions, or even to report on their own understanding and comprehension. This can make education and learning evaluation much more difficult.

Communication and Cultural Considerations

COMMUNICATION SKILLS THAT IMPACT THE INTERVIEW PROCESS

When a patient is in significant pain, sufficient to bring them to a health care provider, it is important to utilize **effective communication skills** in order to successfully work around the profound distraction of the pain. Patients observe nonverbal behaviors as a health care provider works with, assesses and interviews them. The interviewer should always appear calm and unhurried, regardless of time constraints. Condescending tones of voice or behaviors must not be used, and the interviewer must avoid making judgments and/or stereotyping patients. Greet the patient using their formal name unless or until asked otherwise. Use eye contact, appropriate personal space, and a warm tone of voice and touch to encourage an atmosphere of trust and acceptance. In this way the individual is best prepared to provide accurate, timely information.

COMMUNICATION AND ITS RELATIONSHIP TO PAIN

Communication is a process that is transactional (on the same level) and reciprocal (mutual). Two people must engage to create meaning behind exchanges of information. Messages are generated, sent and received. The true importance is not in the message that is sent but rather in the manner in which it is perceived. **Pain expression** is impacted by many factors, one of which is the difficulty encountered in communicating that pain perception. Patients who can articulate their discomfort clearly and are able to openly ask for pain management (either medicinal or otherwise) are more successful in obtaining pain control than those who cannot effectively communicate their pain. Thus, communication is vital to successful pain management and individuals who cannot communicate that pain for whatever reason are likely to suffer.

THERAPEUTIC RELATIONSHIP

A relationship between the patient and nurse commences when the nurse begins to provide care and the patient accepts that care. Unlike other legal relationships there is no written contractual agreement. However, the nurse is held to a formal legal standard of care. With regard to pain management, nurses should know that all persons have the right to pain control, and withholding that care can lead to legal difficulty. A **therapeutic relationship** is one in which the nurse provides expert care to the patient in a manner that fosters safety, confidentiality and honesty. No stereotyping or judgment is passed, and a patient is taken at their word and is presumed to be providing accurate and honest reports in return. The quality of the therapeutic relationship can significantly impact the care that the patient receives, and therefore may greatly influence the patient's health outcomes.

BARRIERS TO COMMUNICATION

Many factors can become **barriers to communication**, including language, culture, and visual and hearing deficits, to name a few. Overcoming these barriers is vital to meaningful communication and therefore to the treatment of the individual. Interpreters may be used to communicate when language is a significant barrier. Caution, however, must be exercised to ensure that the interpreter does not have beliefs and values that may color or influence the interpretation and communication process. Using visual aids or written materials in the patient's native language may be helpful without introducing bias. Utilizing different devices and mechanisms (e.g., patient-controlled analgesia, or PCA device) may enhance communication because of the increased sense of confidence and control introduced by the use of the machine. Information gathered from the PCA itself could also help communicate pain needs as well.

PAIN EXPRESSION AS RELATED TO CULTURE

Culture deeply affects the expression and perception of pain as well as an individual's ability and likelihood of communicating about pain to others, including health care providers. Pain perceived by the physical body usually results in an effective response, but the specific pain expression will often be influenced by culture and background. Two broad categories of expression have been identified: stoic or emotive. They may be described as follows:

- **Stoic** – represented by the patient who either "grins and bears it" (i.e., tries to project an image that all is well) or who does not outwardly express any acknowledgement of their pain (i.e., they are often silent in their suffering).
- **Emotive** – represented by the patient who is verbally expressive of their pain. This patient may moan and cry out in seeking outward expression of their pain.

PATIENT ADVOCACY

Nurses have an obligation to investigate all methods that may decrease a patient's pain. Anything within the scope of nursing practice that is safe, effective, and applicable to pain management should be tried. This includes but is not limited to: pharmacologic options, non-pharmacologic methods, holistic and spiritual supports, technology advances that may be appropriate, and any noninvasive therapies. The use pain management delivery equipment (epidurals, PCA devices, etc.) is not a substitute for the acknowledgement of pain, or for the nurse's presence in the pain management process. The concept of advocacy implies an adversary or entity that is either neglectful or acting against the best interests of the patient. Thus, the nurse must be insistent upon pain control with every patient.

To be a successful **pain control advocate**, several principles must be integrated into nursing practice. First, nurses must recognize pain. It is sometimes easy to unwittingly overlook the pain that another person is facing. Nursing is a busy, hectic profession and the nurse may not always realize the pain a patient is experiencing. However, to be an effective patient advocate, pain must never be ignored. Indeed, it must be actively sought out. Take each patient's pain seriously, recognizing when it may be necessary to disturb a physician, even at times after midnight, to report uncontrolled pain and request appropriate orders. Be an active advocate for that patient. Always empathize with patients, and do not judge. Trust that they are in pain when they state it as a fact. Finally, a nurse must be willing to educate themselves past the point of generic pain control information offered in traditional nursing education if they wish to be a skilled pain control advocate.

Ethics

American Nurses Association Code for Nurses

The following are components of the **American Nurses Association Code for Nurses established in 1985**.

1. The nurse provides services with respect for human dignity and the uniqueness of the client unrestricted by considerations of social or economic status, personal attributes, or the nature of health problems.
2. The nurse safeguards the client's right to privacy by judiciously protecting information of a confidential nature.
3. The nurse acts to safeguard the client and the public when health care and safety are affected by the incompetent, unethical or illegal practice of any person.
4. The nurse assumes responsibility and accountability for individual nursing judgments and actions.
5. The nurse maintains competence in nursing.

Self-Determination and Pain Control

Autonomy is one of the major concepts governing pain management in the health care system. Autonomy is medically defined as "a patient's right to **self-determination** regarding health care," and it may affect pain control on many levels. Therefore, all individuals have a right to make decisions that impact their lives, and thus their course of treatment, in a time of ill health and/or crisis. This means that patients must also be involved in decisions regarding pain control and the related interventions employed on their behalf. The result is that patient self-determination may significantly alter the pain treatment process. It is important to note that pain management and the side effects that that accompany treatment will affect different people in different ways and to differing degrees. Thus, a patient's wish, particularly when based on past experience, may sometimes differ from what is expected.

Informed Consent and Pain Treatment

Informed consent is based on the principle that a patient has the right to accept or reject proposed treatments based upon complete information explained in a manner that is understandable. The acting physician has the responsibility of obtaining informed consent. The following elements must be included to obtain true informed consent.

- An explanation of the diagnosis, disease or condition that warrants treatment.
- The nature and purpose of the treatment, explained in appropriate language.
- The potential and probable outcome if treatment is not pursued.
- The benefits and material risks of the proposed treatment.
- Any reasonable alternative treatments, including their inherent material risks and benefits.
- Finally, the probability of success of the treatment should be explained.

INFORMED CONSENT, PATIENT EDUCATION, AND SELF-DETERMINATION IN REGARDS TO PAIN CONTROL

Obtaining **informed consent for pain control therapies** is a cornerstone in the process of self-determination and the right of individuals to make decisions that determine the course of their lives, and thus their health care. There are informed consent guidelines pertaining to what information a patient is to receive before authorizing a procedure. Patients should always be provided with ample education and information before any decisions are made or consent forms are signed. Teaching about pain, pain management therapies, risks and benefits, and the availability of alternatives and options should always take place. Also, discussions regarding any cultural or religious beliefs or feelings regarding the meaning of pain should be taken into consideration, so that self-determination and informed consent are truly authentic.

PLACEBO AND PLACEBO EFFECT

A **placebo** is an intervention or medication that has no therapeutic effect, but which the patient believes to be efficacious. Placebos are used for their symbolic effect or to eliminate observer bias in controlled research experiments.

The **placebo effect** is defined as a change in the patient's condition that is attributed to the administered placebo, regardless of whether the placebo was a pseudo-procedure, pseudo-medication, or any other symbolic form of medical therapy. Therefore, the change in condition is attributed to the symbolic effect of the placebo and not the actual action taken.

The **effectiveness of placebo interventions** varies according to the intervention and surrounding circumstances. There are a multitude of factors that have an impact on a patient's response to placebo therapy. The concept of the placebo effect is important, however, especially in the context of the patient-physician relationship. It has been shown that a placebo is often more effective in treating a patient than no treatment at all. The placebo effect may be caused by a release of endorphins that impact current symptoms, or the patient may report a positive response so that the patient-physician therapeutic relationship will remain stable and they will continue to get help. Patients rely on physicians to provide helpful, effective medicinal treatments, and that reliance may contribute to the success of placebos as well.

SIDE EFFECTS

Placebos, even with their inherent inert nature, are not without **side effects.** Placebo treatments may cause drowsiness, headaches, nervousness, nausea, constipation or insomnia. Placebo treatments have also been found to alter laboratory results and other physiological measurements. There are nonspecific impacts of some placebo treatments that may produce nocebo effects: adverse effects caused by negative expectations surrounding the prescribed treatment. There is also a learning process to consider. Aversive conditioning takes place when negative results are associated with treatments patients have received in the past. This learning process or conditioning may affect current and/or future treatments that are intended to decrease real pain. Because the placebo effect is documented and powerful, it follows that side effects of placebo use are real and can be detrimental to the patient and the future treatment of their pain.

OPPOSING ARGUMENTS

A major **argument against placebo use** is based on the concept of true informed consent. Informed consent is impossible to obtain when placebo therapies are used. The principles of fidelity (responsibility to keep one's promises) and veracity (duty to tell the truth and avoid deception) are both violated by the use of placebo treatments. Placebo use is admonished by the American Society of Pain Management Nurses, the American Medical Association's Code of Medical Ethics, and the American Nurses Association Code for Nurses as well. The Joint Commission also stipulates that a patient's rights are violated by placebo use.

ARGUMENTS FOR PLACEBO USE

There is some belief that, because of the strength of the placebo effect, some placebo therapies can be used therapeutically without deception of the patient. The belief hinges on the ability of health care providers to use non-deceptive means to encourage the use and effectiveness of placebos in their patients. Arguments for such use of placebos also assert that every encounter of the patient and the health care provider in a therapeutic setting will provoke an additional placebo effect. This argument is based on the idea that there is an expectation of comfort and caring between a patient and nurse, and that these expectations will further relieve their symptoms. All these factors work together to produce positive outcomes for placebo interventions, whether they were intended as placebo therapies or not.

BIASES

There are many **barriers created by biases** held by health care providers. A nurse can knowingly or unknowingly hold a bias against a patient for their race, gender, socioeconomic background, religion or culture. These beliefs can hinder nursing care in general and pain management in particular, if the nurse allows these hidden biases to affect their treatment of the patient's pain. A nurse must openly accept all pain reports from the patient. Pain should be defined as what the patient reports it to be. No judgments or bias should be allowed to interfere with the treatment of a patient's report of pain.

Certainly, the health care worker can be afflicted by bias and judgments that inhibit or prohibit adequate and effective management of pain in a patient. However, the **biases of a patient** can also become a significant factor in the successful treatment of pain. Many patients have preconceived beliefs and ideas regarding pain control, and about the methods and therapies associated with such treatments. Many of these patients are under-treated for pain because of their own misconceptions regarding the risk of addiction to opioid therapies. Patients can also hold biases regarding the appropriateness of reporting their pain, sometimes believing that a stoic demeanor is the proper approach to dealing with pain. Other patients may have developed an innate distrust of the health care system, perhaps because of past inadequate care, and the therapies offered therein. These biases will need to be overcome to provide effective pain relief treatment.

OPIOPHOBIA

Opiophobia is defined as the fear of opioid therapy and the risk of addiction accompanying its use. Patients can be under-treated for pain when their own opiophobia prohibits them from accepting appropriate pain management. Opiophobia can also be a professional fear that hinders the appropriate therapeutic administration of opioids by the nurse or prescribing physician. A nurse may also under-treat a patient based on fears of respiratory depression, a potentially real but manageable side effect of opioid therapy. In some scenarios, administering opioid medications can also hasten death. The potential for that outcome can be too significant for some health care providers, and their resultant fears may prevent them from administering opioid medications even in appropriate circumstances.

Confidentiality

Confidentiality in the treatment of patients with pain is an important part of the health care provider's responsibilities. No information regarding the therapeutic use of opioid therapy should be shared in any manner outside of communication within the health care system to facilitate a continuum of care. As with any patient, the details and facts of the pain management patient's health and wellbeing belong to them alone, and they have the right to confidentiality and the dispersal of that information to only those individuals who are authorized and involved in their medical treatment. As a health care worker, confidentiality should be an integral part of daily practice.

Responsibility Regarding Abuse and Addiction

Health care providers are as likely as anyone else to fall victim to **substance abuse** and the disease of drug and alcohol addiction. However, health care providers also work within a system that continuously exposes them to these substances. Every health care provider has a legal and ethical responsibility to uphold the law and, within the scope of their practice, to protect society from drug abuse and addiction. Health care providers also have the responsibility to dispense medication to those who need it and to protect that same medication (through protocol and proper procedures) from those for whom it is not intended. Nurses should educate themselves on agency policies and protocols for the use and administration of controlled substances. This is the best way to avoid drug diversion and protect the profession and practice.

Drug Abuse by Health Care Providers

Health care workers may exhibit **unique symptoms of drug abuse** or addiction because of the unique environment in which they work. The following behaviors may be linked with drug abuse and/or addiction:

- Excessive absenteeism or inappropriately long breaks.
- Unexplained long absences.
- Lingering at the medication portal.
- Inappropriately timed and lengthy bathroom visits.

All are possible signs of a problem. Health care workers who are struggling with drug abuse/addiction may also often volunteer for overtime or show up at work when not scheduled. These same individuals may be unreliable in keeping appointments or have difficulty meeting scheduled deadlines. Finally, they may exhibit high and low periods of productivity and/or an unusual number of mistakes due to inattention, poor judgment and bad choices.

A **potentially addicted health care** worker may:

- Take an inappropriate length of time to complete routine tasks.
- Become easily confused or forgetful.
- Have difficulty concentrating and following directions or tasks.
- Be reluctant to admit responsibility for errors or mistakes.
- Their relationships with coworkers may suffer.

There may also be heavy wasting of drugs, drug shortages and/or sloppy documentation. Their appearance, hygiene, demeanor and work may show a rapid and consistent decline, and they may insist on injecting all narcotics themselves. Finally, they may begin to isolate themselves personally and professionally, and complaints about their work and professional performance will increase.

PALLIATIVE CARE

Palliative care is described as treatment rendered with the intent to provide comfort, rather than to cure, arrest or maintain a medical condition. It is most often provided to patients who are at the end stages of life. Palliative care affirms life and considers dying as a normal process. Palliative care is not intended to hasten or postpone death, and is not considered curative treatment of any kind. The focus of palliative care is on relief from pain and other distressing symptoms. Patients have unique psychological and spiritual needs and these are also addressed within the palliative care model. A medical support system is offered with the intention of sustaining and maintaining the patient's ability to live and function as fully as possible until the time of their death. The patient's family is also supported with efforts to help them cope, both during the patient's illness and when encountering the experience of grief.

ISSUES IN PAIN MANAGEMENT AS END-OF-LIFE APPROACHES

Pain can change rapidly and the characteristics and qualities of pain can change significantly as well, as **end-stage of a disease** approaches. It may sometimes even include a decrease in pain, possibly from reduced hepatic or renal function which may extend the metabolic half-life of analgesics being used to treat pain. There may also be co-morbid factors (i.e., hypercalcemia) that may decrease the sensation of pain. However, an increase in pain may also occur due to rapid disease progression and the increasing number and frequency of treatments used to address the disease and its symptoms. Often, in evaluating end-of-life pain, it is less important to decipher the origin of any pain as much as to promptly relieve it. Pain at this stage is less "fixable," and diagnostic tests and procedures may be unrealistic at this point.

PAIN MANAGEMENT IN THE END-OF-LIFE STAGE

Pain management in a patient who is not imminently dying is dealt with very differently from that of a patient who is actively nearing the end of their life. The risks to the patient must be weighed more carefully against the benefits, as their tenuous health status frequently makes the risks greater. Also, time is increasingly crucial. Often there is not time to try different pain control methods and tediously evaluate success. Instead, pain control must be achieved promptly, and the risks must be weighed in the bigger picture of end-of-life goals. Research shows that 85 percent to 90 percent of cancer patients can achieve good analgesia, if the World Health Organization cancer pain ladder is employed. Patients who do not obtain good pain control through traditional approaches should be receiving all other alternate methods available until they secure adequate pain relief.

QUALITY OF LIFE IN THE DYING PATIENT

Dealing with **patients and families who are nearing the end of life** can be challenging and uncomfortable. People confronting death often have different definitions of what quality of life means to them, particularly as it may be defined by their loved ones who are still well. The following factors have been found more meaningful to dying patients and should be thoughtfully addressed:

- **Dignity:** Not becoming a burden, and continuing to be valued.
- **Resilience:** A patient's ability to withstand stress and maintain emotional control.
- **Malaise:** Lethargy, somnolence, and generally not feeling well.

- **A sense of connection:** Patients want people with them who are intimately important to them, and they do not want to feel alone.
- **Sense of closure:** The patient wants to have said and done all those things that are important, ensuring that they leave no loose ends.
- **Spiritual wellbeing:** Patients want to have spiritual and/or philosophical meaning to their lives.
- **Transcendence:** To prepare for the loss of one's physical body.
- **Suffering:** Patients do not want to suffer pain, anguish, terror or hopelessness.

Documentation Requirements

DOCUMENTATION AS A LEGAL DOCUMENT

Documentation completed by nursing staff can be one of the most effective and reliable ways for communication to occur between caregivers. Any documentation recorded for the purpose of medical records is considered a legal document and can be subpoenaed in cases involving legal action. Not only does the nurse hold the responsibility to provide pain treatments as prescribed, but also to document within the standard of care regarding the safety and efficacy of prescribed treatments. Documentation should include the patient's history, assessment, and care plan, as well as interventions used and a regular evaluation of pain levels and subsequent analgesic treatments provided. All documentation should be detailed, concise and complete. Well recorded nursing notes will serve to protect the nurse and the agency if subsequent legal action were to occur.

APPROPRIATE PATIENT INFORMATION TO DOCUMENT
PATIENT INFORMATION AND PATIENT ASSESSMENT

In **documenting a patient's personal information and pain management therapy,** it is appropriate to record a patient's name, age, and diagnosis, as well as any allergies, significant medical history (including chemical dependence), the reason they are seeking pain management (surgery, cancer, acute injury, etc.) and any instructions given to the family and/or patient.

When a patient is receiving opioid administration, documentation of vital signs, pain rating and sedation level are all required if the medication is delivered by one or more of the following routes: buccal, transdermal, rectal, parenteral or oral. All patients receiving intraspinal analgesia necessitate further assessment including: level of sedation, sensory level, motor level and the condition of the epidural site, if applicable.

PAIN MANAGEMENT

Documentation involving a patient receiving pain management therapy includes many requirements. Patients receiving opioid analgesia should be closely monitored and all findings recorded completely. Nursing interventions are often employed as complimentary adjunct to medicinal or medical interventions. These adjunctive interventions should be documented in as precise a manner as any other medical procedure, including the specific intervention, the pain rating before and after, and the response and willingness of the patient to try the technique again, as well as any teaching that occurred for the patient and/or family. Evaluation of the pain management plan should take regularly place, including: real or potential adverse effects, either medicinal or nursing interventions involved, as well as an evaluation of the effectiveness of the utilized pain interventions.

Opioid Administration and Use

Administration of opioid medications, including their use and their waste, involve specific highly controlled documentation. Monitoring of the dosage of opioid medication administered should include specific documentation of that information, as well. When opioids are being administered by infusion devices (patient-controlled analgesia or epidural, etc.) then documentation of the cumulative doses that are received every three to four hours must also to be documented. Every agency has a protocol for the disposal and waste of residual opioids that are contained in infusion bags or are otherwise rendered unusable. Specific protocols should be followed as well as documented completely every time opioid medication is wasted. This is done to protect the health care providers from possible suspicion of inappropriate opioid use.

Substance Abuse

Among other unique considerations, when **treating a patient who has a known substance abuse history** documentation of accurate and specific facts is essential. Documentation of medicinal pain management therapy should include several specific parameters. The amount of drug dispensed should recorded as well as any specific instructions and teaching provided. Accurately document the date the medication was given to the patient as well as noting which pharmacy is designated to fill the prescription. Include a pharmacy printout of any prescriptions the patient has received as well as the prescriber identification number with the Drug Enforcement Agency (DEA). Any pharmacological effects of the analgesia should be documented, in addition to any side effects. Any ancillary interactions with the patient also should be recorded, including visits and phone calls.

Opioid Medication in the Home Health Care Setting

Specific legal protocols need to be initiated and maintained during **opioid therapy in the home health care setting**. Opioids need to have safe storage (particularly in homes with small children or family members with known/documented drug abuse issues). This storage needs to be documented and communicated to other involved case workers. Complete records regarding opioid administration must be maintained, along with documentation of the proper disposal of opioids administered by intravenous, rectal, oral or transdermal routes. Be sure to also document patient and caregiver instructions concerning opioid administration, including any possible adverse effects, a determined course of action for breakthrough pain, and any emergency plans of action that may be needed. Appropriate disposal of all sharps should also be documented in this setting.

Fentanyl Patches Used in the Home Health Care Setting

Fentanyl patches should be applied, per order, and should include the date and time applied on the patch itself. Each nursing shift in the home health care setting should document that the patch was checked and that both the dose and integrity of the patch were verified. Disposal of fentanyl patches in the home health care setting will include further documentation. Disposing of or wasting any fentanyl patches must be documented by two nurses' signatures. Because the home health care setting presents unique concerns regarding the use of opioid therapy, complete, accurate and astute documentation must promptly take place to protect the health care provider and to ensure the safety of the patients.

Long-Term Opioid Therapy

Documentation concerns for varying medical scenarios have different requirements. When documenting **long-term opioid therapy** with a patient experiencing nonmalignant pain, the following should be included in the report: An intake assessment including pain assessment, a history and physical examination, chemical use and abuse (both past and present), and any support systems that are in place, as well as the individual's living situation. Random, periodic urine screenings are common throughout treatment and these results should be included in the documentation. As treatment continues, ongoing assessments should continue to take place. At each interaction with the patient, the pain level should be ascertained as well as any side effects they are experiencing. Their physical and psychosocial functioning should be recorded, as well as the development of any maladaptive drug-related behaviors.

DOCUMENTATION NEEDED TO APPROPRIATELY PRESCRIBE CONTROLLED SUBSTANCES

A **physician** must accurately document a number of issues and points of information before safely prescribing controlled substances to any patient. These include:

- A medical history and physical examination should be completed, regardless if one exists from a referring physician. The medical history should include information regarding any past treatments of pain, any history of substance abuse, and the effects of any past pain experience on physical and psychological functioning. Finally, a diagnosis that is in appropriate for prescribing controlled substances must be entered in the medical record.
- Further documentation should be entered as periodic reassessment of the patient is made, particularly highlighting patient progress toward established treatment goals.
- A treatment plan should be written and included in the documentation. An outline of therapeutic treatments and changes in treatment should also be included. Outcomes should be identified as markers for treatment success are accomplished (i.e. improved ability to function within activities of daily living, etc.).

Additional information that a physician must document when prescribing controlled substances includes:

- Referrals to other physicians or consultants should be noted.
- A relationship with the patient's pharmacist should be ongoing and documented. The patient should be receiving controlled substances from only one pharmacy/pharmacist, as well as Scheduled drugs being prescribed by only one physician if at all possible.
- Any addictive behavior should be assessed on a continuous basis with documentation of the findings these assessments. It may become necessary for a physician and patient to draw up a contract outlining appropriate behaviors and responsibilities on the part of the patient in order to continue receiving prescriptions for controlled substances.
- There should be written evidence that the risks, benefits and alternatives to narcotics were discussed with the patient.
- Documentation must also outline the failure of any non-narcotic medications previously given, justifying the current need for narcotic options.

Standards of Care

ASPMN STANDARDS OF CARE

The **American Society of Pain Management Nurses (ASPMN)** has provided nurses with standards of care. They are divided into six standards that affect and guide the assessment, planning, intervention and evaluation of chronic pain patients by the nursing team:

- **Standard I – Assessment.** A systematic evaluation and comprehensive communication of the patient's experience of pain, their symptoms or other pain-related information should take place. This information should then be interpreted back to the patient and again with the health care team.

- **Standard II – Problem Focus/Diagnosis.** An evaluation of the complete assessment data should take place. Any and all problems should be identified as well as their impact on the plan of care.
- **Standard III – Outcome Identification.** Clinical outcomes (realistic goals) should be identified between the health care provider and patient. These outcomes should evolve throughout the continuum of care.
- **Standard IV – Planning.** The health care team should then develop a comprehensive pain management plan based upon the previous steps.
- **Standard V – Implementation.** Facilitation and implementation of identified pain management strategies should begin.
- **Standard VI – Evaluation.** Responses to the pain management plan, the implemented pain management strategies, and any forward movement toward identified outcomes (goals) should be evaluated and documented.

ANA Standards of Care

The **American Nurses Association (ANA)** provided these standards of professional performance for nurses in 1991.

- **Quality of care.** The nurse should systematically evaluate the quality and effectiveness of the nursing practice. The nurse should participate in quality care activities that are appropriate and timely to his or her position, education and practice setting. Also, the nurse should guide changes in practice with information learned through the quality of care activities. The nurse should also aim to make changes throughout the health care delivery system based on information garnered from the quality of care exercises. Nurses have the potential and ability to be significant change agents for the patients they work with, their own practice, those who practice around them, and for the entire health care delivery system.

ANA Code for Nurses

The following are **six further components** of the American Nurses Association Code for Nurses established in 1985.

- The nurse exercises informed judgment and uses individual competence and qualifications as criteria in seeking consultation, accepting responsibilities and delegating nursing activities to others.
- The nurse participates in activities that contribute to the ongoing development of the profession's body of knowledge.
- The nurse participates in the profession's efforts to implement and improve standards of nursing
- The nurse participates in the profession's efforts to establish and maintain conditions of employment conducive to high-quality nursing care.
- The nurse participates in the profession's effort to protect the public from misinformation and misrepresentation and to maintain the integrity of nursing.
- The nurse collaborates with members of the health care professions and other citizens in promoting national efforts to meet the health care needs of the public.

Joint Commission Standards for Pain Management

The **Joint Commission** has provided health care practitioners with standards of care for pain management. They are as follows:

- Health care workers should involve patients in all aspects of their care, including but not limited to effective pain management.
- Patients have the right to adequate assessment and treatment of their pain.
- Pain should be assessed in all patients. It is to be considered the fifth vital sign behind blood pressure, heart rate, temperature, and respirations.
- There are established policies and procedures that will support the safe prescription or ordering of medications, including scheduled prescriptions, and patient-controlled analgesia. Spinal administration of medications and other pain management technologies should be used appropriately in the care of patients with pain.

The **Joint Commission** has provided health care providers with further standards of care for pain management. They are as follows:

- After a procedure, the patient is to be monitored for pain intensity, duration, location, character and responsiveness to treatments. Other parameters should be considered as well.
- Patient education regarding pain and the management of pain is to take place as appropriate and needed.
- At the time of discharge, the planning process should provide information for the patient's assessed needs at the time of discharge. Symptom management (i.e. pain) is to be included.
- The organization is to collect regular performance information in an ongoing effort to monitor its adherence to accreditation standards, including appropriateness and effectiveness of pain management.

APS Quality of Care Committee

The **Quality of Care Committee** recommends that an interdisciplinary team be organized to analyze the process of pain management and evaluate any deficits in care. The recommendation is that, at the minimum, one member of the team must have specialized pain management experience. Meetings should be scheduled as needed, with an expectation of meetings held at least every three months, to review pain management processes and outcomes. Where advanced technologies are used, the team should assess any complications and adverse effects. Clinical units should work with the team to establish procedures to improve pain management. The quality improvement team should report to administration, medical, nursing and pharmacy staffs about their learning and any new recommendations.

Standards of Care

The **American Pain Society (APS)** has established a Quality of Care Committee to provide recommended standards of care in the management of pain. The committee states that pain is to be recognized and treated promptly. Health care providers should document and also display the patient's report on the pain experience. There are several key variables that typically affect the pain process, and these variables should be continually improved upon. Health care staff should document outcomes based upon the information gathered, and provide prompt feedback to those who need it. Information about analgesics should be readily available to patients along with explicit assurances from staff that they will be attentive to their pain control needs. There should be explicit policies in place regarding the use of advanced analgesic technologies.

Research and Quality Improvement

NURSING RESEARCH

Nursing research is a process of accumulating new knowledge through a systematic process. The knowledge acquired can be new information, an enhancement of known information, or an expansion of existing knowledge. This information contributes to the practice of nursing. Nursing research helps to build professionalism for nurses as well as providing them with evidence-based practice guidelines. Nursing research also helps provide accountability to patients, health care agencies, third-party payers (insurance companies) and health care workers. As the health care arena changes, nursing research helps to show the efficacy of nursing and the positive impact on its patients. The process of nursing research expands our knowledge base in many ways and provides many enduring benefits.

QUANTITATIVE RESEARCH

Quantitative research is the collection of numeric data through a reliable, ordered process. The conditions of the data collection and analysis are carefully controlled. Quantitative research uses statistical processes to manipulate data in order to illustrate and describe certain phenomena, or to assess the strength and dependability of relationships drawn between two or more variables.

Quantitative correlational studies explore the connections between variables of interest without any active participation or intervention on the part of the researcher (e.g., studying the correlation between gender and various forms of pain responses).

Quasi-experimental studies are designed to examine causality. Because the participants in such a study cannot be randomly assigned specific treatment conditions, these types of studies are subject to questions of validity. To enhance validity the researcher manipulates the independent variables and employs certain controls.

EVALUATION, RESEARCH, NEEDS ASSESSMENT, AND METHODOLOGICAL RESEARCH

Evaluation research is designed to determine how well a program, policy, procedure, practice or protocol is working. A needs assessment is a quantitative design constructed similarly to evaluation research. This method is used to provide administrators, decision makers and policy makers with the information they need to take appropriate action. This information assists in the planning process by collecting data to estimate the continuing and future needs of a group, community or organization.

Methodological research refers to controlled investigations regarding how we obtain, organize, analyze, and validate data obtained via other research methods. Research tools are developed, validated and evaluated on their performance by methodological form of research.

EXPERIMENTAL STUDY DESIGNS

Experimental study designs attempt to examine causality by manipulating certain independent variables in order to produce a change in certain dependent variables. Generalizability (an effort to obtain results applicable elsewhere) is obtained by randomly assigning subjects to the planned intervention groups. A control group (receiving no intervention) will also be used for reference point purposes. Key factors in an experimental study design include manipulation, control and randomization. An example of an experimental study might be a postoperative treatment study. A group of postoperative patients are randomly assigned to different treatment modalities (the independent variables to be manipulated). One set of patients will receive oral opioid therapy while the second receives patient controlled analgesia through an intravenous infusion device. The outcome measured (the dependent variable) is satisfaction with pain control. This type of study (randomized clinical trial) is often used in health care studies (e.g., to test new medications, procedures, etc.).

PROCESS OF QUALITATIVE RESEARCH

Qualitative research is the systematic, interactive, subjective process that is used to describe life experiences and provide them with organized meaning. Qualitative research examines concepts and phenomena needing descriptive and narrative clarification. This type of research often generates theories, and hypothesis that are intended to be further quantitatively researched later. Qualitative research uses participants that are purposefully selected because they have specific characteristics in common (e.g., a study regarding the effects of depression on learning would require participants who are depressed and willing to talk (descriptively) about their learning experiences during periods of depression). In this research process the researcher is involved heavily with the participants and uses inductive analysis to identify themes and collected related information. A narrative approach is utilized to report their findings.

DESCRIPTIVE STUDIES

Descriptive studies focus on the precise description of a subject's characteristics, situations, groups, and/or the frequency with which certain events occur. There is no manipulation of the variables in this type of research and a summary will provide central tendency measures such as standard deviations and means.

Typical descriptive studies examine the characteristics of a particular group. An example may be a study of a fibromyalgia population, with

a focus on generating information regarding their lifestyle, sleep habits, health and wellness practices, as well as their employment environment, etc.

Comparative descriptive studies are used to describe differences between two or more groups. For example, one may comparatively study a population of people suffering from fibromyalgia and a population of individuals who are suffering from migraine headaches.

TIME-DIMENSIONAL STUDIES AND CASE STUDIES

Time-dimensional studies are focused on studying progressions and pattern of change and growth as they trend over time. Longitudinal studies look at the changes in the same sample of subjects over an extended period of time. One example would be studying the effect of using a TENS unit on patients with chronic back pain. Cross-sectional design is a time-dimensional research construct that studies groups of sample subjects in various stages of development concurrently. An example of a cross-sectional study would be researching the effects of opioid therapy on two hospitalized populations: patients with a history of chemical abuse longer than ten years and patients with a history of such abuse less than five years.

Case studies examine any number of identified variables as related to a single unit: a person, family, group, community or institution. The goal is to analyze the selected unit based upon a defined set of variables, seeking patterns and themes in the data. This is an intensive and exhaustive exploration process.

PARADIGMS AND LIMITATIONS OF THE RESEARCH PROCESS

A **paradigm** is a construct of an individual's particular perspective, providing a model, pattern, worldview or framework on how the originator believes a specific situation or concept should be perceived. In research, a paradigm will guide how research questions are formulated as well as the methods that the researcher will use to search for answers to the research question.

An **empirical paradigm** posits that there is order, objective, and nonrandom reality to life. A researcher with a natural paradigm will believe that reality is subjective and is mentally constructed by the participants in any individual research studies.

Clearly, research studies have **limitations**. The design and sampling techniques that are used, as well as measurement and data collection are all sources of these limitations. Further, there are always moral and ethical constraints that may limit some of the questions that may be pursued and some kinds of measurement methods, etc. Finally, ensuring complete control in any research environment is not genuinely attainable. A significant limitation is the complexity of human beings and how they impose themselves (and thereby influence) on any research undertaken.

CLINICAL RELEVANCE AND POTENTIAL OF NEW RESEARCH FOR IMPLEMENTATION

In determining the **clinical relevance of new knowledge**, it important to decide if a significant problem will be eliminated by applying the new intervention or by changing the existing practice. If the answer is yes, the research has clinical relevance. In determining the information gained by research and its potential for implementation one must look at transferability: Is it appropriate for the new innovation to be tried in a different setting? Are there enough staff, resources, along with a fertile organizational climate, including external resources and the potential for clinical evaluation to warrant the use of the new intervention? (i.e., is it feasible?) As always, a cost-benefit ratio should be calculated and taken into account when deciding whether or not to implement a new innovation.

USE OF NURSING RESEARCH AND BARRIERS TO RESEARCH BEING USED

Nursing research becomes useful when it serves to influence or alter existing practices and nursing protocols. There are many factors that can create barriers to the use of knowledge that is gathered through nursing research. For example, if the research is insubstantial (i.e., if there is a lack of knowledge that has been accrued by valid, reliable research studies or a shortage of comparable studies that have been reported), then the knowledge will likely not be put into practice. If the organization itself lacks resources to disperse the information, or they are resistant to change, then the information can remain sequestered. With nursing professionals, there can be difficulty between the researcher and other clinicians and their beliefs that hinder adequate research utilization. Finally, if the information cannot be communicated easily or there are other institutional roadblocks to the research, the knowledge may not be put to use.

QUALITY IMPROVEMENT

The process of **quality improvement** for pain control nurses is governed by the standards of care provided for the nursing profession by the American Nurses Association (ANA), the Joint Commission, the American Pain Society (APS), and the American Society of Pain Management Nurses (ASPMN). These standards of care are based on research and are considered evidence-based practice. The continual process of nursing research and quality improvement will steadfastly influence, revise and alter the standards of care as warranted by the newly generated knowledge. Nurses involved with the pain management of patients are responsible for knowing and adhering to these evolving standards of care and being aware of changes that occur.

Important Terms

Culture—A set of beliefs, values, and practices shared by a group or community of people. Learned behaviors are passed down from older generations to younger ones.

Ethnicity—Belonging to a particular ethnic group. An ethnic group shares characteristics like race, language, religion, values, symbols, literature, folklore, music, food, settlement patterns, employment patterns and common geographic origin.

Ethnocentrism—Believing that the best way to behave, believe and conduct oneself is according to one's own culture. Believing that one's own culture is superior to all others.

Stereotyping—When assumptions are made about all people of a particular race, ethnic background, or who share some other common demographic feature. Stereotypes persist when no learning takes place to confirm or dispel these conceptions/misconceptions.

Generalization—Inferring specific traits in a person, group, circumstance, or entity based upon prior broad observations or experiences. This is considered a beginning point and more information about a particular individual should be accumulated before conclusions regarding this unique individual can be made.

Acculturation—A process by which a smaller cultural group begins to take on the behaviors, values and life-ways of a more dominant culture. The smaller culture's traditions, behaviors, values and life-ways can become extinct.

Assimilation—When an individual or group incorporates specific selected characteristics of another culture without taking on all of the attributes of the dominant (or larger) cultural group.

Autonomy—Refers to a patient's right to self-determination. Patients should make their own, informed choices regarding their health care whenever possible.

Beneficence—Is the commitment to do good and avoid harm.

Nonmaleficence—Refers to the duty to do no harm.

Justice—Refers to the principles of fairness, impartial treatment and high-quality equitable care for all patients regardless of race, ethnicity or diagnoses. It also includes the fair distribution of health care resources to all patients.

Veracity—Refers to the duty to tell the truth, and to avoid lies and deception.

Fidelity—Refers to strict adherence to one's duties, responsibilities and promises.

Euthanasia—The purposeful administration of a treatment intended to cause death in the case of a patient for whom death is deemed beneficial. Sometimes referred to as active euthanasia.

Voluntary Active Euthanasia—Euthanasia initiated at the explicit request of a patient deemed competent.

Involuntary Euthanasia—Euthanasia initiated despite the patient's explicit objection.

Non-Voluntary Euthanasia—Euthanasia of a person (either a child or an adult) who lacks the capacity or the ability to consent or refuse.

Physician-Assisted Suicide—A physician provides a patient with information or a drug (or both) knowing in advance of the patient's intention to initiate an act of suicide.

Assisted Suicide—When medical provisions (medicines, devices, etc.) or physical assistance are provided to an individual with the knowledge that the person intends to commit suicide.

Quality assurance—Quality assurance is the process of focusing on the delivery of an excellent product. It includes the establishment of a process that ensures the successful delivery of the desired product excellence.

Total quality management—Total quality management addresses the need for continuous and persistent improvements in the processes that provide service and care.

Continuous quality management (CQI)—Continuous quality management (CQI) focuses on the key actions of an organization with the belief that quality is improved by such a focus. CQI focuses on coordinating efforts within the agency and collecting reliable data through effective performance measures. Processes that affect patient care and patient outcomes are also addressed. The theory behind CQI is that instead of looking for a few poor examples of care, one should focus on the continuous opportunities to improve the processes that deliver care.

Grounded theories—Theories that are purposefully developed around the collection, coding, and sorting of data regarding the specific events or concepts being examined.

Ethnography—A research construct designed to examine the culture and/or attributes of a specific people. An emic approach (investigation of a culture from within the culture) or an etic approach (examining the similarities and differences across the culture from outside the culture) may be used.

Historical research—Historical research looks for patterns and relationships from events in the past in a methodical way.

Philosophical research—Philosophical research endeavors to illuminate meanings, make values manifest, identify ethics, and study the nature of knowledge.

Content analysis—Content analysis is a type of qualitative research that provides researchers with an organized, efficient way to measure the frequency, order and/or intensity derived from the occurrence of words, phrases or sentences in processes of communication, because of their importance to a theoretical postulation.

Pain Management Nursing Practice Test

1. Balanced analgesia refers to:
    a. providing the patient with patient-controlled analgesia.
    b. providing analgesia PRN when the patient requests it.
    c. using two or more forms of analgesia concurrently.
    d. administering analgesia at preset time periods.

2. The pain management nurse should educate a mother who states she is giving her 4-year-old child aspirin to relieve muscle aches associated with the flu because:
    a. aspirin doesn't adequately relieve discomfort.
    b. aspirin may cause Reye's syndrome.
    c. aspirin may make the symptoms of flu worse.
    d. acetaminophen is more effective.

3. The pain management nurse makes an effort to always act for the good of the patient. This is an example of the ethical principle of:
    a. autonomy.
    b. nonmaleficence.
    c. integrity.
    d. beneficence.

4. A 28-year-old patient with three young children has ovarian cancer and is to be discharged to her home with fentanyl transdermal patches for pain control. When teaching the patient about the use of the patches, the pain management nurse should stress that discarded patches:
    a. must be immediately flushed down the toilet.
    b. can be discarded into any waste basket.
    c. should be cut into small pieces before discarding.
    d. can be discarded in any manner as they are harmless.

5. A patient experiences a traumatic injury and the external stimulus converts into an electrical signal that the patient can perceive as pain. This is an example of:
    a. modulation.
    b. perception.
    c. transduction.
    d. transmission.

6. Which of the following statements by a patient indicates that the pain management nurse needs to provide education?
    a. "I take all kinds of herbal medicines because I know they're always safe."
    b. "I stopped eating grapefruit because it interacts with so many medications."
    c. "I always try to look up the side effects of medicines I'm taking."
    d. "I take acetaminophen for headache instead of NSAIDs or aspirin."

7. An older adult has received an opioid for pain but has developed some confusion as a result. The patient, hearing a siren, insists that a woman is screaming. The best response is:
   a. "That sound is nothing to worry about."
   b. "That sound is an ambulance siren."
   c. "Don't worry, we'll help the person."
   d. "She'll stop screaming in just a minute."

8. As team leader, the pain management nurse must work collaboratively with a number of team members. When the pain management nurse is delegating a task, the delegation process should begin with:
   a. specific timeline for completion of the task.
   b. identification of necessary resources.
   c. identification of priorities.
   d. the task to be delegated and the expected outcomes.

9. The theory of pain that states that pain is produced by the brain and spinal cord and not damage to the tissues and that different parts of the CNS work together to create the perception of pain is the:
   a. Cartesian theory.
   b. Gate keeper theory.
   c. Neuromatrix theory.
   d. Specificity theory.

10. According to the WHO three-step ladder approach to pain management, if a patient's abdominal pain associated with pancreatic cancer varies from 4 to 8 on the pain scale, pain control should be initiated at
   a. step 1.
   b. step 2.
   c. step 3.
   d. whichever step is appropriate at the time of initiation.

11. A patient's friend is visiting and expresses concern about the patient and asks for an update on the patient's prognosis. The pain management nurse should:
   a. provide a general update about the patient without going into detail.
   b. tell the visitor it's not appropriate to ask for information about the patient.
   c. tell the visitor the pain management nurse cannot discuss the patient's condition.
   d. deny knowledge of the patient's prognosis.

12. If a pain management nurse makes derogatory statements about a patient to a third party, the nurse may be liable for:
   a. libel.
   b. slander.
   c. assault.
   d. battery.

13. A patient with chronic low back pain states he wants to try complementary therapy to relieve pain as medications have been ineffective and asks the pain management nurse which of the therapies are most likely to relieve discomfort. The pain management nurse should reply that therapy that has documented effectiveness is:

   a. acupuncture.
   b. herbal medicines.
   c. homeopathic medicines.
   d. healing touch.

14. According to the American Pain Society's guideline for the use of chronic opioid therapy for chronic non-cancer pain, the factor that most indicates a risk of drug abuse or misuse after beginning chronic opioid therapy is:

   a. severe pain.
   b. older age.
   c. preexisting cognitive impairment.
   d. personal/family history of substance abuse.

15. Which of the following is characteristic of nociceptive pain?

   a. Acute aching or throbbing pain localized to the site of injury.
   b. Diffuse or cramping pain.
   c. Association with chronic conditions, such as diabetes or cancer.
   d. Burning, stabbing, or shooting pains.

16. A common cause of complex regional pain syndrome is:

   a. chronic/repetitive overuse.
   b. depression/anxiety.
   c. crushing injury.
   d. systemic lupus erythematosus.

17. The 5 key elements of pain assessment include (1) words, (2) intensity, (3) location, (4) duration, and (5):

   a. method/administration
   b. aggravating/alleviating factors.
   c. frequency.
   d. quality.

18. A 69-year-old patient with severe cognitive impairment has fallen and fractured her elbow. Which if the following pain assessment methods is most appropriate?

   a. PAINAD.
   b. FACES.
   c. 1-10 scale.
   d. LANSS.

19. Tricyclic antidepressants increase the levels of which neurotransmitter(s)?

   a. Dopamine.
   b. Acetylcholine.
   c. Acetylcholine and glutamate.
   d. Serotonin and epinephrine.

20. Which of the following disorders has a pain pathology associated with sensory hypersensitivity?
   a. Post-herpetic neuralgia.
   b. Rheumatoid arthritis.
   c. Fibromyalgia.
   d. Gout.

21. If a patient receives an antibiotic injection and mistakenly believes it is an analgesic and reports that it has relieved pain, the most likely reason is:
   a. the patient didn't have pain.
   b. the placebo effect relieved the pain.
   c. the pain has simply subsided.
   d. the patient wants attention.

22. When collaborating with a patient and family in developing the plan of care, it's important for the patient and family to understand:
   a. their rights and responsibilities.
   b. their limitations.
   c. the organization's philosophy.
   d. the difference between goals and objectives.

23. If a patient is prescribed extended-release morphine (Kadian®, Avinza®), the pain management nurse must caution the patient to avoid:
   a. grapefruit juice.
   b. exercise.
   c. high-fat foods.
   d. alcohol.

24. A hospice patient who has been taking oral morphine to control the pain of pancreatic cancer reports little relief of constant pain, so the patient is to receive ketamine to relieve pain along with lorazepam once or twice daily in addition to the opioid. When ketamine is administered parenterally, the dosage of the opioid should:
   a. be reduced by 25 to 50%.
   b. remain unchanged.
   c. be increased by 25%.
   d. be increased by 50%.

25. A hospice patient asks if the pain management nurse or doctor can give her an overdose to cause her death because she is tired of suffering pain. The most appropriate initial response is:
   a. "It's illegal for nurses and doctors to give overdoses to cause death."
   b. "You don't really mean that!"
   c. "Let's work together to better control your pain."
   d. "You should talk to the doctor about that."

26. The principle of the double effect refers to the idea that:

   a. drugs may not be used to control pain if they hasten death.
   b. drugs may be used to control pain even if they hasten death.
   c. drugs should not be administered in order to hasten death.
   d. drugs can be administered in order to hasten death.

27. Which of the following opioid drugs should be avoided for pain control in children?

   a. Codeine.
   b. Hydromorphone.
   c. Morphine sulfate.
   d. Fentanyl.

28. Which of the following drugs is most likely to provide relief of pain with intermittent claudication associated with peripheral artery disease?

   a. Statin.
   b. Antihypertensive.
   c. P2Y12 inhibitor (clopidogrel).
   d. Platelet-aggregation inhibitor (Cilostazol).

29. A patient has developed tolerance to morphine sulfate and is to undergo opioid conversion to a different drug. The first step in opioid conversion is to:

   a. use an equianalgesic table to determine the correct dose.
   b. determine total dosage of analgesia in previous 24 hours.
   c. increase the dosage of new drug over current dosage.
   d. stop the current analgesia for 12 hours.

30. A patient is receiving Reiki massage as adjunctive therapy to promote relaxation and reduce stress and anxiety. Reiki massage is classified as a(n):

   a. whole medical system.
   b. mind-body therapy.
   c. energy therapy.
   d. bioelectromagnetic therapy.

31. A patient with chronic osteoarthritis in the left knee complains of mild to moderate pain and stiffness. The initial treatment regimen should begin with:

   a. NSAIDS.
   b. acetaminophen.
   c. hyaluronidase injection.
   d. opioid.

32. A patient has severe pain from envenomation of a pit viper (rattlesnake) while awaiting treatment with antivenin. Which pain control method is most appropriate?

   a. Morphine.
   b. NSAID.
   c. Warm compress.
   d. Ice pack.

33. A patient with pancreatic cancer is switching from oral opioids to transdermal fentanyl patches for round-the-clock pain control. Before applying the patch, skin preparation includes:
   a. cleansing skin with alcohol wipe.
   b. washing skin with soap and water.
   c. shaving hair at site.
   d. clipping hair at site.

34. A 30-year-old patient complains of post-operative pain at 8 on a 1 to 10 scale 12 hours after abdominal surgery although the patient is not moaning, grimacing, or exhibiting signs of pain. The patient last received pain medication 6 hours earlier and has orders for morphine every 4 hours as needed and ibuprofen every 6 hours as needed. Which is the most appropriate action?
   a. Give ibuprofen.
   b. Give morphine.
   c. Give ibuprofen and if no relief in one hour give morphine.
   d. Question family members present about the patient's pain tolerance before making a decision.

35. Which of the following is a recommended treatment (American Academy of Neurology) to relieve pain associated with post-herpetic neuralgia?
   a. Capsaicin (topical).
   b. Morphine.
   c. Gabapentin.
   d. Methylprednisolone (epidural).

36. Which of the following is an example of a violation of professional boundaries?
   a. The nurse assists the patient to make a telephone call.
   b. The nurse accepts a gift of candy to be shared by all staff members in the unit.
   c. The nurse pats the patient's arm to show support.
   d. The nurse confides in the patient that the nurse is distressed because the nurse's mother is ill.

37. A 10-year-old girl with juvenile idiopathic arthritis has severe pain and stiffness in the morning upon awakening. Which of the following interventions is likely to provide the best relief?
   a. Using an electric blanket for 10 minutes before arising.
   b. Doing active range-of-motion exercises before arising.
   c. Taking aspirin each morning 30 minutes before arising.
   d. Taking a corticosteroid each morning 30 minutes before arising.

38. A 20-year-old female patient reports having 4 to 6 severe unilateral throbbing headaches monthly with each lasting 4 to 72 hours and accompanied by nausea, photophobia, and phonophobia. Exercise and strenuous activity (such as stair climbing) increases the intensity of the headaches. These symptoms are characteristic of which type of headache?
   a. Cluster headache.
   b. Episodic migraine.
   c. Tension-type headache (TTH).
   d. Secondary headache.

39. A 62-year-old female with increasing diffuse soft tissue pain but without joint swelling over the past 6 months as well as frequent headaches and difficulty sleeping is diagnosed with fibromyalgia. The pain management nurse focuses initial treatment for pain on:

    a. pregabalin, duloxetine, or milnacipran.
    b. NSAIDs, antiepileptic drugs, duloxetine.
    c. NSAIDs, other analgesics, complementary therapy.
    d. CBT, relaxation exercises, and lifestyle modifications.

40. A patient with stage 4 prostate cancer has recently completed a course of radiation to relieve spinal compression from bone metastasis. His pain is well controlled with fentanyl, but he is fearful and he has developed tremors and jerking movements of his extremities, and these are keeping him awake at night. The pain management nurse recognizes that the most likely cause of the tremor and jerking movements is:

    a. brain metastasis.
    b. spinal damage.
    c. anxiety.
    d. opioid-induced myoclonus.

41. The most important factor in ensuring compliance with the treatment regimen is:

    a. education.
    b. follow-up.
    c. therapeutic relationship.
    d. cost.

42. Drug absorption may be impaired in gerontology patients because of:

    a. decreased splanchnic (visceral) blood flow.
    b. body water volume fluctuations.
    c. decreased renal blood flow.
    d. changed hepatic volume.

43. According to DEA regulations for Schedule II drugs, what is the refill limitation without renewal by a healthcare practitioner?

    a. 0 refills.
    b. 2 refills.
    c. 5 refills.
    d. 12 refills.

44. When doing medication reconciliation for a geriatric patient, the pain management nurse is concerned that some medications or dosages may be inappropriate for older patients. The most efficient method of checking these medications is probably to consult:

    a. *Physicians' Desk Reference* (PDR).
    b. *Drugs.com*.
    c. Beers Criteria.
    d. drug manufacturers.

45. Which of the following drugs is generally most effective for treatment of trigeminal neuralgia?

   a. Baclofen.
   b. Phenytoin.
   c. Gabapentin.
   d. Carbamazepine.

46. If a patient who is addicted to narcotic drugs undergoes a surgical procedure and complains of postoperative pain, the patient should receive:

   a. non-narcotic analgesia only.
   b. analgesia appropriate to the type and degree of pain.
   c. minimal doses of opioid analgesia.
   d. maximum doses of opioid analgesia.

47. If a Hispanic patient shows non-verbal indications of pain (tense, withdrawn, frowning, holding her chest) as well as increased respiratory and heart rate but describes pain on a 1-to-10 scale as "two," the pain management nurse should:

   a. assume the patient is not in acute pain.
   b. ask the patient about pain in another way.
   c. assume the patient is stoic and simply denying pain.
   d. explain the 1 to 10 scale again.

48. A Christian Scientist patient with advanced cancer steadfastly refuses pain medications because of religious beliefs. The best approach for the pain medication nurse is to:

   a. try to reason with the patient about pain medications.
   b. stop working with the patient.
   c. explore alternative/complementary therapies with the patient.
   d. try to convince the patient's family to intervene.

49. Which of the following statements by a patient indicates the need for education?

   a. "Pain is just a natural part of aging."
   b. "Pain should be controlled so that is bearable."
   c. "Healthcare providers should take my pain seriously."
   d. "I have the right to make decisions about treatment for pain."

50. According to the CHEOPS pain scale, which of the following combinations of symptoms may indicate that a 1-year old infant is in pain after surgery?

   a. Neutral facial expression, random movements of lower extremities.
   b. Whimpering, restless movement of legs.
   c. Inactive, not touching or reaching toward incision.
   d. Not crying, inactive, random movements of lower extremities.

51. A patient had surgical repair of a knee but over time instead of the pain in the surgical site lessoning, it worsened. This type of pain is referred to as:

   a. allodynia.
   b. hypoalgesia.
   c. secondary hyperalgesia.
   d. primary hyperalgesia.

52. Which of the following is an example of therapeutic communication?
 a. "Don't worry. Everything will be fine."
 b. "You should listen to your doctor."
 c. "Is there anything you'd like to talk about?"
 d. "Why are you so upset?"

53. When using music therapy to help a patient relax, the most important criterion is:
 a. genre of music.
 b. patient preference.
 c. delivery system.
 d. rhythm and beat.

54. After a patient receives morphine for pain, which of the following symptoms is most cause for concern?
 a. Patient develops moderate myoclonus (twitching).
 b. Patient's respirations slow from 20 to 16 per minute.
 c. Patient falls into a deep sleep.
 d. Patient appears lethargic.

55. A patient taking high doses of opioids has had persistent constipation but complains of a sudden episode of diarrhea and increasing urinary incontinence. The most likely cause is:
 a. enteritis.
 b. fecal impaction.
 c. allergic response to medication.
 d. malabsorption syndrome.

56. Which type of neuropathic pain occurs with herpes zoster?
 a. Polyneuropathy.
 b. Deafferentation.
 c. Mononeuropathy.
 d. Sympathetically-mediated.

57. Which type of pain most often requires opioids to control?
 a. Visceral.
 b. Neuropathic.
 c. Somatic.
 d. Psychological.

58. A patient has been self-medicating with 2000 mg of acetaminophen every 3 to 4 hours around the clock for back pain, believing it to be free of adverse effects; however, the patient has developed acetaminophen toxicity. The recommended reversal agent is:
 a. naloxone.
 b. flumazenil.
 c. vitamin K.
 d. N-acetylcysteine.

59. A patient tells the pain management nurse that she is barely having any pain and rarely takes pain medications, but her pain medication record shows she has been averaging about 20 to 25 mg of hydrocodone daily. This probably indicates that:

   a. the patient is actively lying.
   b. the patient is reluctant to admit the degree of pain.
   c. the patient is giving the medication to someone else.
   d. the patient is confused.

60. Which pain scale is most appropriate for use with an 8-year old child who has suffered a traumatic injury?

   a. CRIES.
   b. FACES (Wong-Baker).
   c. 0-10 pain intensity scale.
   d. CHEOPS.

61. A patient receiving morphine experiences severe respiratory depression. Which medication is indicated to control symptoms?

   a. Flumazenil.
   b. N-acetylcysteine.
   c. Neostigmine.
   d. Naloxone.

62. Examples of Schedule IV drugs include:

   a. marijuana, heroin, and LSD.
   b. pregabalin and centrally-acting antidiarrheals with atropine (Lomotil®).
   c. benzodiazepines and tramadol.
   d. cocaine, morphine, and fentanyl.

63. Which of the following adjuvant analgesics is most indicated to relieve pain associated with spinal cord compression?

   a. Pamidronate.
   b. Clonazepam.
   c. Nifedipine.
   d. Prednisone.

64. A palliative care patient is receiving chemotherapy through a port in the upper chest but complains that the needle insertion is very painful, so she becomes very anxious before treatment. Which therapy is most indicated?

   a. EMLA cream.
   b. Extra pain medication.
   c. Relaxation exercises.
   d. Anti-anxiety medication.

65. A patient who abruptly stops an opioid after radiotherapy shrinks a tumor and then exhibits withdrawal symptoms has probably developed:

   a. addiction.
   b. tolerance.
   c. physical dependence.
   d. pseudoaddiction.

66. If a patient receives 10 mg of morphine, what is the equianalgesic dose of hydromorphone?

   a. 50 mcg.
   b. 1.5 mg.
   c. 7.5 mg.
   d. 130 mg.

67. Based on general cultural differences, which ethnic group tends to be the least expressive when in pain?

   a. Asians.
   b. Hispanics.
   c. Middle Easterners.
   d. Southern European/Mediterranean.

68. A patient is using a 72-hour fentanyl patch to relieve pain and has good pain control for 48 hours but routinely experiences increased pain for the last 24 hours. The best solution is to:

   a. increase the dosage or change the patch more frequently.
   b. change to a different drug.
   c. use complementary therapies, such as acupuncture.
   d. increase the use of oral opioids for the last 24 hours.

69. The opioid medication that is most likely to cause pruritis is:

   a. oxymorphone.
   b. fentanyl.
   c. codeine.
   d. morphine.

70. The federal law that gives patients the right to make decisions about care based on informed consent and to accept or refuse treatment is the:

   a. *American's with Disabilities Act* (ADA).
   b. *Emergency Medical Treatment and Labor Act* (EMTALA).
   c. *Patient Self Determination Act* (PSDA).
   d. *Health Insurance Portability and Accountability Act* (HIPAA).

71. A pain management nurse monitoring pain control for a patient with a history of drug abuse is concerned that the patient is exhibiting aberrant drug-taking behavior. Which of the following is of most concern?

   a. The nurse finds a rolled and partially burned fentanyl patch beside the patient's bed.
   b. The patient took one extra dose of oral pain medication.
   c. The patient changed his fentanyl patch in 2 days instead of 3.
   d. The patient complains that he needs higher doses of medication.

72. In the ABCDE method of pain assessment, the E stands for:

   a. eliminate pain.
   b. empower patients and family.
   c. expectations.
   d. examine patient.

73. Non-steroidal antiinflammatory drugs (NSAIDs) are contraindicated as co-adjuvants with which of the following?

   a. Anticonvulsants.
   b. Corticosteroids.
   c. Bisphosphonates.
   d. Antidepressants.

74. Which of the following is a conditional risk factor for substance abuse?

   a. An unstable home environment.
   b. Poor sense of self-esteem.
   c. Mental health disorder, such as schizophrenia.
   d. Association with members of gangs.

75. Which adjuvant drug is most appropriate for osteolytic bone pain?

   a. Tricyclic antidepressants.
   b. Anticonvulsants.
   c. Corticosteroids.
   d. Bisphosphonates.

76. A patient's pain has been well controlled with morphine sulfate, extended release, but she has developed severe side effects and is being switched to an equianalgesic drug. The dosage of the new drug should be:

   a. equianalgesic dose.
   b. 25% above equianalgesic dose.
   c. 10% below equianalgesic dose.
   d. 25% to 50% below equianalgesic dose.

77. A patient with ovarian cancer is receiving a starting dose of parenteral morphine 5 mg every 4 hours around the clock to control pain but has required 5 rescue doses of supplementary opioids during the past 24 hours. The best action is to:

   a. increase baseline opioid dose.
   b. change to a different opioid.
   c. institute opioid rotation.
   d. add adjuvant medications.

78. Distraction as a pain management tool is most effective for:

   a. severe, acute pain.
   b. chronic pain.
   c. short periods of acute discomfort.
   d. neuropathic pain.

79. Which of the following ECG findings indicates a patient considered for methadone treatment may be at increased risk of ventricular tachycardia or cardiac arrest with the drug?

   a. Occasional PVCs.
   b. 0.5 mm ST elevation.
   c. QTc <450 ms.
   d. QTc >450 ms.

80. Patients with constant severe pain should receive pain medication:
   a. when pain breaks through.
   b. on demand.
   c. routinely around the clock.
   d. four times daily.

81. A patient with an implanted pacemaker has persistent low-back pain and asks the pain management nurse about using a TENS machine that a friend loaned the patient. The pain management nurse should advise the patient:
   a. the TENS machine is safe to use with a pacemaker.
   b. the TENS machine is contraindicated with a pacemaker.
   c. the TENS machine should only be used below the waist.
   d. the TENS machine should only be used at low settings.

82. The pain management nurse is teaching a patient to manage her pain pump for patient-controlled analgesia (PCA). Although the pain management nurse explains at least 3 times, the patient asks the same questions over and over. The pain management nurse provides a pamphlet with illustrations, but the patient barely looks at them and states she can't figure out what she needs to do. The next best approach is probably to:
   a. suggest a different method of pain control.
   b. arrange for someone else to manage the equipment.
   c. allow a rest period and then start again with instructions.
   d. allow the patient to practice with actual equipment.

83. When doing a heel prick or blood draw on a young infant, which of the following usually provides the best pain relief?
   a. Non-nutritive sucking with pacifier.
   b. Sucking with pacifier dipped in 24% sucrose.
   c. Caressing the infant.
   d. Holding the infant.

84. To effectively use guided imagery and visualization as a relaxation technique to reduce anxiety and pain, the child should generally be:
   a. over 4 years old.
   b. over 6 years old.
   c. over 10 years old.
   d. over 12 years old.

85. According to Krasner's Chronic Wound Pain Experience (CWPE) model, what intervention would be specifically instituted to relieve cyclic acute wound pain?
   a. Transcutaneous nerve stimulation.
   b. Tri-cycle antidepressants.
   c. Soaking dressing to loosen prior to removal.
   d. Application of heat.

86. A patient with bone cancer has been reluctant to take adequate analgesia because it conflicts with his self-image as a stoic, strong, active man, but the pain restricts his functional abilities, leading to depression and anxiety. The best approach for the pain management nurse is to focus on how pain medication can:
   a. relieve pain.
   b. reduce depression.
   c. reduce anxiety.
   d. increase functional abilities.

87. When using a lidocaine soak to prevent pain during debridement of an ulcer, how long should the soak be in contact with the wound before beginning debridement?
   a. 3 to 5 minutes.
   b. 10 to 15 minutes.
   c. 20 minutes.
   d. 30 minutes.

88. If morphine is administered subcutaneously, when does the peak analgesia occur?
   a. In 5 to 10 minutes.
   b. In 20 minutes.
   c. In 30 to 60 minutes.
   d. In 50 to 90 minutes.

89. A patient has second-degree burns on both hands with blistering and sloughing of outer layers of skin. Which initial pain control method is generally preferred?
   a. IV morphine.
   b. Transdermal fentanyl patch.
   c. Oral hydrocodone.
   d. Soaking hands in ice water.

90. If using the PQRST method of pain assessment, an appropriate question to begin the assessment with is:
   a. "Does the pain move or stay in one place?"
   b. "When did the pain start?"
   c. "What causes the pain?"
   d. "What does the pain feel like?"

91. Which position is usually best to relieve acute low back pain?
   a. Side-lying curled position with knees and hips flexed and pillow separating knees.
   b. Sitting upright in a soft chair.
   c. Standing at a walker with weight supported by extending arms.
   d. Lying prone.

92. In reviewing a patient's records, the pain management nurse notes that the patient's pain seems poorly controlled when under the care of one particular nurse, but that nurse has documented that the patient receives the medication every 4 hours as prescribed. The pain management nurse should suspect:
   a. the nurse causes the patient increased stress.
   b. the patient's pain level naturally fluctuates.
   c. the patient is developing tolerance.
   d. the nurse is diverting the patient's medication.

93. When applying an ice pack to a patient's lower back to relieve pain, what is the maximum duration of time the ice pack should be left in place?
   a. 10 minutes.
   b. 20 minutes.
   c. 30 minutes.
   d. 45 minutes.

94. The primary treatment for moderate to severe cancer-related pain is:
   a. NSAIDs.
   b. complementary therapy.
   c. opioids.
   d. acetaminophen.

95. According to the Pain Care Bill of Rights, patients have the right to:
   a. have pain thoroughly assessed and treated.
   b. be free of pain.
   c. take opioids for the relief of pain.
   d. have all pain interventions covered by insurance.

96. A patient with Guillain-Barré syndrome reports severe pain but the patient's facial expression has remained unchanged. This probably indicates:
   a. exaggerated report of pain.
   b. depression.
   c. flaccid facial paralysis.
   d. stoic reaction to pain.

97. The cause of post mastectomy pain syndrome is:
   a. psychological stress.
   b. swelling and edema.
   c. metastasis.
   d. direct damage to the nerves.

98. When using diclofenac sodium 1% gel for relief of joint pain, the patient should ensure the right dosage by:
   a. using a teaspoon measure.
   b. using the dosing card/ruler.
   c. estimating the correct amount.
   d. applying small amounts and increasing until pain controlled.

99. The Gate Control Theory of Pain explains why pain:
   a. is sometimes blocked and other times not.
   b. is focused at the site of injury.
   c. is controlled by the brain.
   d. is primarily subjective.

100. A 22-year-old patient returning from war with a traumatic BK amputation of his left arm has phantom pain that has been unrelieved by opioids, antidepressants, anticonvulsants, and nerve stimulation. Which of the following interventions is the most appropriate to try next?
   a. Acupuncture.
   b. Brain stimulation.
   c. Mirror box.
   d. Stump revision.

101. Which of the following refers to the direct stimulation by chemical, thermal, or mechanical nociceptors, which results in the transmission of electrical signals along neural pathways?
   a. Somatic pain.
   b. Visceral pain.
   c. Nociceptive pain.
   d. Neuropathic pain.

102. Melzack postulated that information from multiple neural systems integrates and produces the pain experience. Which of the following is the title of Melzack's theory?
   a. Specificity theory.
   b. Neuromatrix model of pain.
   c. Gate control theory.
   d. Pattern theory.

103. Which of the following pain conditions features chronic moderate to severe soft tissue pain and allodynia?
   a. Temporomandibular joint disorder.
   b. Radiculopathy.
   c. Fibromyalgia syndrome.
   d. Peripheral neuropathy.

104. Which of the following statements is accurate regarding the most effective management of cancer pain?
   a. Better education of health-care providers on recommended guidelines for treating pain is essential.
   b. The avoidance of opioid usage is necessary to prevent future addiction problems.
   c. The administration of nonsteroidal anti-inflammatory drugs (NSAIDs) subcutaneously is effective for maximum pain control.
   d. The continuous administration of opioids subcutaneously is an extremely expensive therapy.

105. Central sensitization is of paramount importance in the pathogenesis of chronic pain. The definition of central sensitization is a complex condition in which an increase in the excitability of CNS neurons results in unusual senses and responses to various stimuli. Which of the statements below best describes the dorsal horn mechanism known as hyperalgesia?

   a. An amplified response to painful stimuli.
   b. A progressive increase in the scale of response to C fiber activity.
   c. The concept that cellular memory for pain may lead to future increased responses to nociceptive stimuli.
   d. The development of a situation in which, due to recurring excitement of a neuron, the impulse threshold decreases and the strength of the response increases.

106. A neuroma is an unusual growth area on a damaged nerve ending that is frequently the site of ectopic impulse generation and mechanosensitivity. Which of the following statements describing neuromas is inaccurate?

   a. Neuromas may be very small, making palpation challenging or impossible.
   b. Neuromas ensnared in scar tissue may cause continuous activations (neuroma in continuity).
   c. Neuromas are unable to form after limb amputations.
   d. Neuroma formation may occur on myelinated and unmyelinated nerve fibers.

107. In 2001, the American Nurses Association (ANA) Code for Nurses (Table 12-1) declared that pain management nurses were on the front lines of care for those who are most vulnerable to pain and its undertreatment. According to the ANA, which of the following is not included in creating a caring environment as the cornerstone for effective pain management?

   a Continued assessment of the values of the patient, family, and nurse is essential.
   b. Understanding what pain means to a patient provides insight on how to intervene.
   c. Ethics committees play an important role in ensuring institutional commitment to pain management.
   d. Caring implies attaining as much education as possible.

108. Unresolved pain results in the body's stress response and the release of stress hormones. Which of the following conditions do not occur when pain is unrelieved?

   a. Increased myocardial oxygen consumption.
   b. Bradycardia and fluid retention.
   c. Immunosuppression and increase in deep vein thrombosis.
   d. Increased catabolism.

109. Duty is established when a professional relationship is initiated between the nurse and patient. Which of the following best defines breach of duty?

   a. Failure to evaluate and report epidural injection for signs of infection.
   b. Failure to report addiction to legal authorities.
   c. Administration of opioids for pain.
   d. Failure to employ staff with pain management background.

110. Assessment of acute pain includes determining the location of the pain, a description of the type of pain (in the patient's own words), and an evaluation of the pain intensity and duration. What are some of the tools used to establish the intensity of the pain?

   a. Numeric Pain Intensity Scale and Visual Analog Scale.
   b. McGill Pain Questionnaire.
   c. Pain Outcomes Questionnaire.
   d. Brief Pain Inventory.

111. The Checklist of Nonverbal Pain Indicators (CNP) contains several factors that, when observed, could indicate pain in the nonverbal patient. Which of the following behaviors are not included in the nonverbal pain indicators?

   a. Grimacing, and rubbing.
   b. Sleeping and staring into space.
   c. Bracing and restlessness.
   d. Vocalizations and moaning.

112. The pain management nurse uses various aids for assessing acute pain. What are the desired characteristics of these assessment tools?

   a. Easy to use, in simple English, quick, and documentable.
   b. Complex, covering all aspects of the patient's history and complete physical.
   c. Comprehensive, including laboratory tests, x rays, and magnetic resonance imaging or computerized axial tomography scans.
   d. Simple, user-friendly, quick, providing documentable data, and understandable for patients with different languages and cultures.

113. When the pain management nurse uses the FACES Pain Scale, which of the following is inappropriate in describing the faces?

   a. Hurts very bad.
   b. No pain.
   c. Feels very sad.
   d. Very much pain.

114. An important facet of assessing pain is the patient's ethnicity, because it may influence their pain expression and response. Which of the following statements regarding the effect a patient's ethnicity or culture has on their pain response is inaccurate?

   a. Minorities may be at greater risk for undertreatment of pain.
   b. Ethnicity refers to common language, traditions, origins or social backgrounds.
   c. One's culture has a great influence on a person's reaction and communication regarding pain.
   d. Each person has a unique neurophysiological system of pain perception.

115. Which of the following sentences is an example of the interview technique of assessing pain using the psychosocial behavior known as reflection?

   a. "That's understandable."
   b. Touch the patient's arm, lean forward in your chair, and maintain eye contact.
   c. Repeat the patient's statements to elicit a more detailed description.
   d. "Please explain what you mean."

116. When a patient is physically and mentally competent to self-report pain, the Numeric Pain Intensity Scale (NPI) may be an effective tool for pain assessment. Which of the following patients would not be a candidate for using this type of assessment tool?

 a. Patients with chronic pain.
 b. Patients with rheumatic disease.
 c. Patients with dementia.
 d. Patients with cancer pain.

117. An important component of pain assessment is the determination of associative factors. When interviewing the patient, which questions below would not determine associative factors?

 a. Is the patient constipated?
 b. What makes the pain better?
 c. Does the patient have nausea and vomiting with the pain?
 d. Does the pain cause the patient to lose sleep?

118. Which pain assessment tool below is recommended for use with pediatric patients?

 a. Verbal Descriptive Scale (VDS).
 b. FACES Scale.
 c. Brief Pain Inventory (BPI).
 d. McGill Pain Questionnaire.

119. Multidimensional pain scales measure multiple aspects of the pain experience. Which of the following is not an example of the multidimensional pain scale?

 a. McGill Pain Questionnaire.
 b. Verbal Descriptor Scale (VDS).
 c. Brief Pain Inventory (BPI).
 d. Pain Outcomes Questionnaire.

120. The Opioid Risk Tool (ORT) evaluates the risk of prescribing opioids for pain. Which of the following subjects would be appropriate for this assessment?

 a. Familial or personal history of substance abuse, sexual abuse, or depression.
 b. History of psoriasis.
 c. Familial history of hypertension or high cholesterol.
 d. History of diabetes or heart disease.

121. Several barriers prevent adequate pain treatment. Which of the following is not a common problem (in the U.S.) that contributes to inadequate pain relief?

 a. Lack of education.
 b. Misconceptions.
 c. Inadequate supply of medications.
 d. Attitudinal issues.

122. Many people express concern that opioid analgesics will result in addiction and decrease the patient's life span. The opposite is true. Inadequate pain treatment hastens death by all of the following means EXECPT it:
   a. Increases psychological stress.
   b. Decreases mobility.
   c. Increases oxygen requirements.
   d. Increases immunocompetence.

123. The nonopioid analgesic acetaminophen (APAP) is one of the safest analgesics for chronic mild pain. Which of the following statements regarding acetaminophen is inaccurate?
   a. It is excellent as a "coanalgesic" for chronic severe pain.
   b. It works well for nonspecific musculoskeletal pain.
   c. It decreases inflammation and reduces fever.
   d. Reduce dosage or avoid usage in patients with liver or renal disease and alcohol users.

124. Which of the following best describes nonsteroidal anti-inflammatory drugs (NSAIDs)?
   a. Reduce biosynthesis of prostaglandins, inhibiting the cascade of inflammatory events.
   b. Reduce the pain signal throughout the nervous system.
   c. May be useful when administered by patch or oral transmucosal means.
   d. May cause constipation, itching, headache, dysphoria, sedation, and nausea.

125. Which of the following statements best defines "addiction"?
   a. A state of adaptation in which exposure to a drug stimulates changes that result in a reduction in one or more of the drug's effects over time.
   b. A state of adaptation that is evident by the drug-class-specific withdrawal syndrome, which can be elicited by abrupt cessation.
   c. A primary, chronic, neurobiological disease characterized by a lack of control over drug use, compulsive cravings, and continued use despite harmful effects.
   d. The misconception that the need for increases in dosage of a pain medication is due to tolerance instead of disease progression.

126. Which of the following terms refers to the quantity of blood that is completely free of a drug after a set period?
   a. Clearance.
   b. Elimination.
   c. Enzyme induction.
   d. Biotransformation.

127. Body tissues respond to specific chemical agents in a variety of ways. The chemical (drug) may increase, decrease, or replace certain hormones, enzymes, or metabolic functions. Which of the following terms best describes this response?
   a. Mechanism of action.
   b. Cmax.
   c. Efficacy.
   d. Pharmacodynamics.

128. A patient on an opioid analgesic complains of constipation. Which of the following adverse reactions would this most likely represent?

   a. Overdose or toxicity.
   b. Allergic reaction.
   c. Side effect.
   d. Drug interaction.

129. The use of opioids in combination with an NSAID, COX-2 inhibitor, or acetaminophen produces a "dose-sparing effect." Which of the following describes this technique?

   a. Multimodal analgesia.
   b. Therapeutic drug monitoring.
   c. Pharmacokinetics.
   d. Genetic polymorphism.

130. Which of the following terms refers to a drug that interferes with opioid receptors to displace the opioid, producing a reversal of analgesia?

   a. Steroid.
   b. Antagonist.
   c. Hypnotic.
   d. Anxiolytic.

131. Preemptive analgesia refers to the administration of drugs prior to, or during, surgery for the prevention of postoperative pain. Which of the following best describes the action of preemptive analgesia?

   a. Prevents the establishment of altered central processing of afferent input.
   b. Works on various sites in the nervous system.
   c. Temporarily impedes or takes away a sensation.
   d. Binds to physiological receptors and imitates the regulatory effects of endogenous signaling compounds.

132. Which of the following statements is incorrect regarding patient-controlled anesthesia (PCA)?

   a. PCA is a method of analgesic therapy.
   b. PCA is an analgesic delivery pump.
   c. The Joint Commission and Institute for Safe Medication Practices prohibit PCA by proxy.
   d. PCA may not be used in conjunction with authorized-agent-controlled analgesia (AACA).

133. Which of the following is a disadvantage of the analgesic bolus dose of PCA?

   a. The patient pushes a button to administer the opioid.
   b. It minimizes the accrual of the opioid.
   c. The patient must be awake to administer the medication.
   d. Consecutive doses have a lockout to prevent overdose.

134. The technique of continuous infusion of an opioid with bolus capability prevents a subtherapeutic plasma concentration of the medication. Side effects of this type of PCA dosing can be serious. Which of the following signs or symptoms would not indicate a possibly serious reaction to the opioid?

   a. Urinary retention.
   b. Itching.
   c. Respiratory depression.
   d. Constipation.

135. There are several nonmedical modalities for the treatment of pain. Which of the following are not preventive measures that minimize chronic pain conditions?

   a. Lifestyle changes (diet, exercise, stress management, and correct posture).
   b. Cessation of smoking.
   c. Heat therapy, hydrotherapy, and biofeedback.
   d. Limiting alcohol consumption.

136. Which of the following are goals of patient education regarding pain?

   a. Decrease misunderstandings regarding pain; increase observance to pain regimens.
   b. Emphasize patient-centered care; facilitate effective communication between family and patient.
   c. Instill in the patient the concept that pain is private and should not be discussed with family members.
   d. Improve patient understanding of medical jargon.

137. Low literacy levels present unique problems to the pain management nurse when attempting to educate the patient about pain. What are the techniques for teaching the low literacy patient?

   a. Keep content simple, include essential issues, and use visual cues.
   b. Emphasize important content by beginning and ending with it.
   c. Assess the reading levels of education materials required.
   d. Use the lecture technique.

138. Which of the following includes the best tools for evaluating the patient's understanding of material taught in pain management class?

   a. Test and retest, return demonstration, and repetition of content.
   b. Test knowledge of medical terminology and survey.
   c. Patient's evaluation of educator's teaching style.
   d. Patient's level of participation in group discussions.

139. Which of the following should not be included in guidelines for cancer pain education?

   a. Pain can usually be controlled; there is no benefit to enduring pain.
   b. Patients can learn to describe and measure pain levels.
   c. Morphine and morphine-like drugs may be used.
   d. Medications should be kept by the patient's bed in easy-open containers for quick access.

140. Common teaching errors may prevent the patient from understanding the information. Which of the following is not a teaching error?

   a. Incomplete needs assessment.
   b. Testing and retesting.
   c. Using information that is extremely complex.
   d. Not receiving feedback in order to evaluate comprehension.

141. A nurse pain management educator notices that one of his patients is not making eye contact with him and has not opened the materials provided. The best response should be to:

   a. stop the class immediately and ask the patient if they have the ability to read, understand, and use the information.
   b. speak with the patient in private during a break and evaluate their motivation and readiness level and potential language barriers.
   c. document the pertinent information from the class session.
   d. set goals and objectives with the patient.

142. Which of the following is not a goal of educating the public about pain management?

   a. Increase awareness and knowledge of pain management.
   b. Decrease public misconceptions regarding pain management.
   c. Facilitate access to suitable health care.
   d. Assess individual needs of audience members.

143. The pain management nurse has an initial meeting with a new patient. During the initial interview, the patient states, "I'm a grown man; I should be able to tolerate the pain." This statement is an example of:

   a. myths and misconceptions.
   b. literacy problem.
   c. socioeconomic status.
   d. educational level.

144. Adults with low health literacy have unique problems dealing with pain management. Which of the following are examples of difficulties these patients may experience?

   a. They are less likely to correctly follow instructions, may fail to seek preventative care, and may have difficulty understanding how to use the health care system.
   b. They are more likely to make medication errors and misunderstand medication labels.
   c. They are more likely to have inadequate pain relief when using medication properly.
   d. A and B.

145. Which of the following areas is not included in the documentation of the educational session?

   a. Content provided in the session.
   b. Outcomes of the education, if the patient understands and can demonstrate the skill.
   c. The next step in the education plan.
   d. The patient's spiritual beliefs.

146. **A lecture with the addition of computer presentations, slides, videos, teleconferencing, handouts, or Web-based education is known as which of the following teaching methods?**

   a. Clinical practicum.
   b. Didactic.
   c. Andragogy.
   d. Pedagogy.

147. **Which of the following is not included in the standards of practice for the pain management nurse, as these standards apply to education?**

   a. Provide education for the patient and family.
   b. Teach ancillary personnel specific and appropriate aspects of pain management.
   c. Mentor or serve as a resource for nurses with limited pain management knowledge.
   d. Take courses to remain up to date every five years.

148. **Mental illness, anxiety, grief, and cultural and language differences are all examples of:**

   a. common errors in teaching.
   b. patient and family barriers to education.
   c. professional barriers to education.
   d. systemic barriers to education.

149. **Which of the following is not included in the core content of a professional education for the pain management nurse?**

   a. Neurophysiology and pathophysiology of pain and assessment of pain.
   b. Psychosocial aspects of care, spiritual aspects of pain, and taxonomy.
   c. Prescriptive authority and prescription writing skills.
   d. Pharmacological and nonpharmacological interventions and common pain syndromes.

150. **Which of the following motivational, learning, and adherence teaching techniques includes the stages of precontemplation, contemplation, preparation, action, maintenance, and relapse?**

   a. Representational approach.
   b. Pain stages of change model.
   c. Transtheoretical model of change.
   d. Health belief model.

Answer Key and Explanations

1. C: Balanced analgesia refers to using two or more forms of analgesia concurrently, such as using a tricyclic antidepressant (amitriptyline) and an anticonvulsant (gabapentin) or an opioid plus another drug. Using multiple drugs may allow lower dosages of each drug so that adverse effects are minimized. Additionally, one drug often potentiates the effects of another drug, providing better control of pain. Balanced analgesia may also delay development of tolerance to opioids because of the lower dosage.

2. B: The pain management nurse should educate a mother who states she is giving her 4-year-old child aspirin to relieve muscle aches associated with the flu because aspirin may cause Reye's syndrome in children with a viral infection, such as chicken pox or the flu. Reye's syndrome can result in swelling of the liver and brain and death. NSAIDs also carry some risk. Young children usually first exhibit diarrhea and dyspnea and older children/adolescents vomiting and lethargy, progressing to confusion, irrational behavior, and seizures.

3. D: If the pain management nurse makes and effort to always act for the good of the patient, this is an example of the ethical principle of <u>beneficence.</u> While it is not always possible to prevent all harm (such as adverse effects of analgesics) to a patient, acting to minimize or avoid harm reflects <u>nonmaleficence.</u> Basing the care of patients on moral standards and being honest with others reflects <u>integrity</u>. <u>Autonomy</u> is the patient's right to self-determination.

4. A: If a 28-year-old patient with three young children has ovarian cancer and is to be discharged to her home with fentanyl transdermal patches for pain control, when teaching the patient about the use of the patches, the pain management nurse should stress that discarded patches must be folded and immediately flushed down the toilet. Used patches still contain the opioid and can result in overdose and death of small children who come in contact with them and are a grave risk to drug seekers who smoke discarded patches.

5. C: <u>Transduction</u> occurs when an external stimulus converts into an electrical signal that the patient can perceive as pain. Transduction is an essential element in the perception of nociceptive pain and facilitates the sense of taste, touch, sight, and hearing. The signal is carried by neurons through <u>transmission</u> up the spinal cord to the brain. <u>Perception</u> of the signal occurs at the cerebral cortex in the brain. <u>Modulation</u> occurs when the body stimulates inhibitory responses.

6. A: The statement by a patient that indicates that the pain management nurse needs to provide education is: "I take all kinds of herbal medicines because I know they're always safe." The pain management nurse should advise the patient that herbal medicines can interact with prescribed medicines, so the patient should always discuss herbal medicines with healthcare providers before taking them and be sure to follow directions regarding recommended dosages. Additionally, some herbal preparations can cause serious adverse effects.

7. B: If an older adult has received and opioid for pain but has developed some confusion as a result; and the patient, hearing a siren, insists that a woman is screaming, the best response is the one that orients the patient to what is real: "That sound is an ambulance siren." It's important not to enter into a debate with the patient (such as when the patient continues to insist on something that is not real/true) but to provide calm support.

8. D: When the pain management nurse is delegating a task, the delegation process should begin with the task to be delegated and the expected outcomes. The pain management nurse should identify priorities if a number of steps or tasks are involved and advise the other team members of monitoring that the pain management nurse may carry out as well as any specific time frame that may be necessary for completion of the task. The team members should be aware of reporting parameters, such as critical information that must be reported immediately.

9. C: The neuromatrix theory of pain states that pain is produced by the brain and spinal cord and not damage to the tissues and that different parts of the CNS work together to create the perception of pain. Because of this, perceptions of pain may vary. For example, if a patient is tense and believes that an injury is severe, the patient may experience pain more severely than if the patient believes the injury is minor.

10. D: According to the WHO three-step ladder, pain control should be initiated at whichever step is most appropriate for the level of pain at the time and then may later be adjusted to a higher or lower step

Level 1	Mild pain	Pain management usually begins with acetaminophen or aspirin followed by NSAIDS well as adjuvant drugs.
Level 2	Mild-Moderate pain	Aspirin or acetaminophen is given WITH codeine and adjuvants. Medications include hydrocodone, oxycodone, and tramadol.
Level 3	Moderate-severe pain	Opioid drugs (morphine, fentanyl, oxycodone)/ Some non-opioid drugs and adjuvant drugs may also be used.

11. C: If a patient's friend is visiting and expresses concern about the patient and asks for an update on the patient's prognosis, the pain management nurse should tell the visitor the pain management cannot discuss the patient's condition. Doing so would be a HIPAA violation. The pain management nurse can only discuss a patient's condition with a parent/caregiver of a minor child, a spouse, or a person with the patient's power of attorney without permission from the patient.

12. B: If a pain management nurse makes derogatory statements about a patient to a third party, the nurse may be liable for slander. If the derogatory statement is in written form, then the nurse may be liable for libel. Assault can be any act that results in the patient feeling fearful (such as threats). If direct harm (such as from abuse or illegal restraint) occurs to the patient, this is battery.

13. A: If a patient with chronic low back pain states he wants to try complementary therapy to relive pain as medications have been ineffective and asks the pain management nurse which of the therapies are likely to relieve discomfort, the pain management nurse should reply that the therapy that has documented effectiveness is acupuncture. Acupuncture appears to stimulate the production of endorphins. Acupuncture is generally safe and has no adverse effects if done by an experienced practitioner. There is little discomfort involved in treatment.

14. D: According to the American Pain Society's guideline for the use of chronic opioid therapy for chronic non-cancer pain, the factor that most indicates a risk of drug abuse or misuse after beginning chronic opioid therapy is personal/family history of substance abuse. Patients with this history should be educated thoroughly about risks and monitored carefully. Other risk factors for abuse or misuse include a younger age and psychiatric comorbidity.

15. A: Nociceptive pain, often described as aching or throbbing, is usually localized to the area of injury and resolves over time as healing takes place and usually responds to analgesia. Nociceptive pain usually correlates with extent and type of injury: the greater the injury, the greater the pain. It may be procedural pain (related to wound manipulation and dressing changes) or surgical pain (related to cutting of tissue). It may also be continuous or cyclic, depending upon the type of injury.

16. C: A common cause of complex regional pain syndrome is a crushing injury. CRPS affects primarily the limbs. Patients many complain of burning, throbbing, cold or heat sensitivity, edema, or changes in skin appearance (pallor, erythema, cyanosis), stiffness, and muscle spasm. Other causes include extended limb immobilization, stroke, sprains, and infection. If not adequately treated, CRPS may progress to muscle atrophy and contractures.

17. B: The 5 key elements of pain assessment include:

- <u>Words:</u> Used to describe pain, such as burning, stabbing, deep, shooting, and sharp. Some may complain of pressure, squeezing, and discomfort rather than pain.
- <u>Intensity:</u> Use of 0-10 scale or other appropriate scale to quantify the degree of pain.
- <u>Location:</u> Where patient indicates pain is located.
- <u>Duration:</u> Constant or comes and goes, breakthrough pain.
- <u>Aggravating/alleviating factors:</u> Those things that increase the intensity of pain and those that relieve the pain.

18. A: If a 69-year-old patient with severe cognitive impairment has fallen and fractured her elbow, the pain assessment method that is most appropriate is PAINAD (Pain Assessment in Advanced Dementia). This scale assesses 5 elements: <u>respirations</u> (hyperventilation, tachypnea, Cheyne-Stokes), <u>vocalization</u> (silence, moan, groan, cry), <u>facial expression</u> (sad, frightened, grimacing), <u>body language</u> (tense, fidgeting, fist clinched, fetal position, combative), and <u>consolability</u> (inability to distract or console).

19. D: Tricyclic antidepressants increase the levels of serotonin and epinephrine by inhibiting their uptake. TCAs serve as antagonists to dopamine and acetylcholine, thus decreasing their levels. Tricyclic antidepressants are lipophilic and highly protein-bound, so they absorb rapidly. TCAs have long half-lives, which increases toxic affects with overdose, and anticholinergic (primarily muscarinic) effects. Because of this, TCAs tend to have more side effects than newer antidepressants: dry mouth, blurring vision, cardiac abnormalities, constipation, urinary retention, and hyperthermia.

20. C: Fibromyalgia has a pain pathology associated with sensory hypersensitivity, which indicates that the cause of the pain cannot be clearly identified. That is, there is no evident damage to nerves or tissue that may account for neuronal dysregulation. Patients often have multiple symptoms and pain in multiple areas of the body. Additionally, patients may be hypersensitive to sensory input (light, heat, sights, smells). Stress may exacerbate pain.

21. B: The placebo affect may occur when a patient's expectations about a drug providing pain relief produce a physiologic release of endorphins that, in fact, relieve pain. The American Society for Pain Management has taken the position that placebos should never be administered to patients in lieu of other analgesics. However, placebos are widely used in drug trials to determine if the effects of a drug are greater than those achieved with a placebo.

22. A: When collaborating with a patient and family in developing the plan of care, it's important for the patient and family to understand their rights and responsibilities. The pain management nurse should ask them what their goals and expectation are and what is most important to them. The pain management nurse may ask the patient and family members to separately list those things that are important to them and then compare and discuss the lists because they may not always be in agreement.

23. D: If a patient is prescribed extended-release morphine (Kadian®, Avinza®), the pain management nurse must caution the patient to avoid alcohol. The alcohol may speed up the metabolism of the drug, leading to an increased rate of release and absorption of the drug into the circulatory system. This can result in a fatal overdose of the drug. Extended-release drugs should never be utilized to initiate opioid treatment but may be considered after the appropriate drug dosage is obtained through administration of immediate-release drugs.

24. A: If a patient is to receive parenteral ketamine to relieve pain along with lorazepam 1 mg once or twice daily in addition to the opioid, the dosage of the opioid should be reduced by 25 to 50% when ketamine is initiated. Ketamine can be administered orally, sublingually, or parenterally. An initial test dose, such as 25 mg, is often given and then the dosage is titrated upward until relief of pain is achieved. If PO or SL, doses may be taken 3 or 4 times daily. Continuous infusions are often used for SC or IV dosing. A number of different protocols are in use.

25. C: If a hospice patient asks if the pain management nurse or doctor can give her an overdose to cause her death because she is tired of suffering pain, the most appropriate initial response is: "Let's work together to better control your pain." Patients who express the desire to die to escape pain often just want to be free of pain rather than really wanting to die, so the patient's pain control should be reviewed and stepped up until pain relief is adequate.

26. B: The principle of the double effect is the idea that drugs may be used to control pain even if they hasten death because the intent is not to cause death but rather to relieve suffering. The Supreme Court (1997) affirmed the principle of the double effect. Most all religions also support the double effect. Patients are usually nearing death when they require such high doses that the drugs may shorten life. In practice, sometimes alleviating pain reduces anxiety and may actually prolong life.

27. A: Codeine is an opioid drug that is generally not recommended for use in children. Meperidine is also not recommended for children for pain control but it may be used to treat shivering. Children may receive morphine sulfate, hydromorphone, fentanyl, hydrocodone, and methadone. Dosage is lower than adults and usually calculated according to kilograms of weight rather than age of child to prevent overdosage.

28. D: While all of these drugs may be prescribed for peripheral artery disease, the platelet-aggregation inhibitor cilostazol is specifically prescribed to relive the pain associated with intermittent claudication. This drug increases blood flow to the extremities; however, it may cause headaches and diarrhea. Pentoxifylline, which has fewer adverse effects, may be prescribed instead of cilostazol, but it is not as effective. If disease is severe, the patient may need surgical angioplasty or a bypass graft in order to get relief of pain.

29. B: Steps to opioid conversion include:

1. Determine the total dose of analgesia during the previous 24 hours.
2. Calculate the equianalgesic dose according to an equianalgesia table.
3. If pain has been controlled, decrease the new medication dosage by 25% to 50% initially.
4. If pain has NOT been controlled, increased the dosage up to 100% to 125% overcurrent equianalgesic dose OR rotate opioids at the equianalgesic dose.
5. Observe patient carefully and titrate dosage up or down during initial 24 hours.
6. Evaluate effectiveness and adverse effects, titrate as needed.
7. Reassess effectiveness of new drug every two to three days.

30. C: If a patient is receiving Reiki massage as adjunct therapy to promote relaxation and reduce stress and anxiety, this treatment is classified as an <u>energy therapy</u>. Energy therapies are intended to affect the aura (energy field) that some believe surrounds living things. Therapeutic touch is also an energy therapy. <u>Mind-body therapy</u> includes support groups, meditation, music, art, and dance therapy. <u>Whole medical systems</u> include homeopathic, naturopathic, acupuncture, and Chinese herbal medications. <u>Bioelectromagnetic therapy</u> uses manipulation of magnetic fields.

31. B: If a patient with chronic osteoarthritis in the left knee complains of mild to moderate pain and stiffness, the initial treatment regimen begins with acetaminophen, which should be limited to 4,000 mg per day because of the risk of liver damage from high doses. NSAIDs should be reserved for more severe pain because of the risks (such as GI hemorrhage) associated with long-term use. If pain persists or condition worsens, the patient may benefit from hyaluronic acid injection or corticosteroid injection into the joint.

32. A: If a patient has severe pain from envenomation of a pit viper (rattlesnake) while awaiting treatment with antivenin, the pain control method that is most appropriate is morphine. Pain is often moderate to severe, and the patient may be very anxious. Ice may further irritate the skin, and heat may hasten the spread of the venom. The patient should receive no aspirin or NSAIDs for at least 2 weeks after the snake bite because of coagulopathy associated with pit viper venom.

33. D: If a patient with pancreatic cancer is switching from oral opioids to transdermal fentanyl patches for round-the-clock pain control, before applying the patch, skin preparation includes clipping hair at the site (avoid shaving, which may irritate skin) and cleansing the skin with water only and allowing the skin to dry completely before application of the patch. No soap, oils, emollients, or alcohol should be used on the skin as these may cause skin irritation or interfere with adherence so that the patch falls off.

34. B: The pain management nurse should give morphine, as 8 on a 1 to 10 scale represents severe pain, not uncommon in the first 24 hours after surgery. Patients have a right to pain control, and the pain management nurse should trust that the pain is what the patient says it is. Patients may show very different behavior when they are in pain. Some may cry and moan with minor pain, and other may exhibit little difference in behavior when truly suffering. Thus, judging pain by behavior alone can lead to the wrong conclusions. Questioning family members is not appropriate.

35. C: Gabapentin is a recommended treatment (American Academy of Neurology) to relieve pain associated with post-herpetic neuralgia. Other recommended treatments include tricyclic antidepressants, lidocaine patch, and opioids; however, morphine is generally ineffective. Capsaicin, epidural methylprednisolone, lorazepam, acupuncture, and laser therapy have also been shown to be ineffective. Some patients receive relief from use of TENS, but others do not. Opioids, such as tramadol and oxycodone, may provide relief for severe pain.

36. D: The nurse must respect and maintain the confidentiality of the patient and family members, but the nurse must also be very careful about disclosing personal information, such as information about a family member, because this establishes a social relationship that interferes with the professional role of the nurse and the boundary between the patient and the nurse. The nurse and patient should never share "secrets." When the nurse divulges personal information, he/she may become vulnerable to the patient, a reversal of roles.

37. A: If a 10-year-old girl with juvenile idiopathic arthritis has severe pain and stiffness in the morning upon awakening, the intervention that is likely to provide the best relief is using an electric blanket for 10 minutes before arising as the heat may relax the muscles and joints. The electric blanket should be set to warm and on a 10-minute timer so that the child is not overheated. Most patients with JIA are already receiving NSAIDS, and corticosteroids are typically used for short periods only because of the risks of adverse effects.

38. B: If a 20-year-old female patient reports having 4 to 6 unilateral throbbing headaches monthly with each lasting 4 to 72 hours and accompanied by nausea, photophobia, and phonophobia, and exercise and strenuous activity (such as stair climbing) increase the intensity of the headaches, these symptoms are characteristic of episodic migraines. Migraines usually have onset in adolescence or early adulthood. The pain is often so severe as to be disabling.

39. D: The pain management nurse focuses initial treatment for fibromyalgia on CBT, relaxation exercises, and lifestyle modifications. CBT helps patients to recognize triggers and to deal more effectively with pain. Patients may need to modify work and should obtain adequate sleep to combat chronic fatigue. Relaxation exercises help patients to cope and reduce stress. Pharmacological agents, such as FDA-approved drugs (pregabalin, duloxetine, and milnacipran), SSRIs, muscle relaxants, NSAIDs, and antiepileptic drugs may provide relief if more conservative treatment is unsuccessful.

40. D: Tremors and jerking movements are consistent with opioid-induced myoclonus, which may be caused by a range of drugs, including opioids and quinolones. In this case, changing to an equianalgesic should relieve symptoms in one to two days. If myoclonus is very mild, a benzodiazepine at bedtime may keep jerking from awakening the patient. While similar symptoms may occur with brain metastasis, it is an uncommon metastasis with prostate cancer. Anxiety may also produce similar symptoms, but less-pronounced and less likely to cause jerking during sleep. Damage to the spine would produce different symptoms.

41. C: While all of these (education, cost, follow-up) are important, the most important factor in ensuring compliance with the treatment regimen is the therapeutic relationship between the patient and the pain management nurse. If the patient feels trust, and the pain management nurse takes the time to discuss patient concerns (such as convenience and cost) and explain both the need for the treatment and the consequences of failing to comply, some of the problems that arise with compliance may be avoided.

42. A: Drug absorption may be impaired in older adults because of decreased splanchnic (visceral) blood flow. Gastric acids tend to decrease and pH tends to become more acidic, and this, combined with decreased blood flow to the stomach, can reduce absorption. Slower gastric emptying can also affect absorption. The degree to which drug absorption may be affected can be difficult to predict although blood levels of some drugs can be monitored.

43. A: According to DEA regulations for Schedule II drugs, no refills are allowed although the healthcare provider may provide a patient for multiple prescriptions for the same Schedule II drug to allow a 90-day supply. However, each prescription must indicate the earliest date by which the patient can fill the prescription. Schedule II drugs include opioids and other drugs that have a high risk of abuse: cocaine, opium, morphine, methadone, Ritalin®, Concerta®, Focalin®, oxycodone, oxymorphone, fentanyl, hydromorphone, hydrocodone (pure), codeine (=/> 90 mg per unit dose), secobarbital, meperidine, pentobarbital, and amphetamine.

44. C: The Beers Criteria (American Geriatric Society) lists drugs that are inappropriate for older adults. The Beers Criteria can be incorporated into clinical decision support systems so that alerts are issued if a medication or dosage is inappropriate for the patient. The Beers Criteria lists the organ system/therapeutic category of the drugs, the rationale for including the drugs on the list, the recommendations (conditions for avoidance and exceptions), the quality and strength of evidence as well as references.

45. D: The most effective treatment of trigeminal neuralgia is generally carbamazepine or oxcarbazepine (although the latter drug is not FDA-approved for this condition). If carbamazepine is not tolerated, then phenytoin, baclofen, lamotrigine, or gabapentin may be tried. Trigeminal neuralgia is characterized by severe stabbing facial pains, aggravated by touch, movement, air movement, and eating. Patients may benefit from Gamma radiosurgery to the trigeminal root or surgical decompression with separation of an anomalous vein from the nerve.

46. B: If a patient who is addicted to narcotic drugs undergoes a surgical procedure and complains of postoperative pain, the patient should receive analgesia appropriate to the type and degree of pain. Even patients who are addicted to narcotics have the right to pain control although they may require larger doses than normal because of tolerance. However, some patients who were formerly addicted may refuse narcotics because of the fear that they will resume drug use.

47. B: If a patient shows non-verbal indications of pain (tense, withdrawn, frowning, holding her chest) as well as increased respiratory and heart rate but describes pain on a 1-to-10 scale as "two," the pain management nurse should ask the patient about pain in another way, such as "mild, moderate, or severe." Although the use of the 1-to-10 scale is ubiquitous in healthcare, it is not commonly used or understood in some cultures, and many people are unsure how to rate pain.

48. C: If a Christian Scientist patient with advanced cancer steadfastly refuses pain medication because of religious beliefs, the best approach for the pain medication nurse it to explore alternative/complementary therapy with the patient. Patients have the right to refuse all medical treatments, including pain medication, and they should not be coerced although the pain medication nurse should explain what options are available to the patient. The patient may, for example, benefit from relaxation exercises and imagery.

49. A: The statement by a patient that indicates the need for education is: "Pain is just a natural part of aging." While it is true that older adults often have pain, that pain always indicates a problem that should be assessed and treated. Aging itself does not cause pain but the chronic diseases, such as osteoarthritis and diabetes mellitus, which are often associated with pain, are more common in the older population, so undergoing routine screenings can help to identify health conditions before they worsen, resulting in pain.

50. B: Whimpering and restless movement of legs indicate pain. Pain ≥4.

Children's Hospital Eastern Ontario Pain Scale (CHEOPS) (Ages 1-7)			
Characteristic	0	1	2
Crying		Not crying	Silent crying, moaning, or whimpering
Facial expression	Smiling, positive	Neutral	Grimacing, negative
Verbalization	Positive, no complaints	Not talking or complaining about other things (not pain).	Complaining about pain or pain and other things.
Torso		Inactive, at rest, relaxed	Tense, moving, shuddering, shivering, and/or sitting upright or restrained.
Upper extremities		Not touching or reaching for wound or injury.	Reaching for, touching gently, or grabbing wound or injury or arms restrained.
Lower extremities		Relaxed, random movement.	Restless or tense moving or legs flexed, kicking crouching, kneeling, or legs restrained.

51. D: If a patient had surgical repair of a knee but over time instead of the pain in the surgical site lessoning, it worsened, this type of pain is referred to as primary hyperalgesia. If the pain involved the surrounding tissues, it would be classified as secondary hyperalgesia. Both types of hyperalgesia may occur after tissue injury and inflammation with increased pain sensitivity. The cause of hyperalgesia is unclear, but it is a type of neuropathic pain.

52. C: "Is there anything you'd like to talk about?" is an open-ended question that encourages the patient to share. Other examples of therapeutic communications are statements that show empathy and observations, such "You are shaking" or "You seem worried," and indicate reality, "That sound is an ambulance siren, not screaming." Pain management nurses should avoid providing advice ("should" or "must") and avoid meaningless clichés, such as "Don't worry. Everything will be fine." Asking for explanations of behavior not directly related to patient care, such as "Why are you so upset?" should also be avoided.

53. B: Music therapy should be tailored to the patient's preference, and this may vary from time to time. For example, a patient may prefer upbeat music during the daytime and quieter music in the evening. While soft classical music is a good general choice, some patients may prefer other genres. Some patients may favor music related to their cultures. The delivery system may vary. In a single room, a radio or music player may be placed by the bed, but in a shared room, the volume should be turned down or the patient fitted with small earphones.

54. A: Myoclonus (twitching) is common after opioid administration and mild twitching is usually not of major concern, but moderate or more pronounced myoclonus may result in seizures. The medication dosage may need to be decreased to control the myoclonus or two or three different medications given in rotation. Respirations of 16 to 20 are both in the range of normal. Lethargy and sleeping often occur with opioids because of their sedative effects and are not cause for concern if patient is otherwise stable.

55. B: Fecal impaction occurs when the hard stool moves into the rectum and becomes a large, dense, immovable mass that cannot be evacuated even with straining, usually as a result of chronic constipation. In addition to abdominal cramps and distention, the person may feel intense rectal pressure and pain accompanied by a sense of urgency to defecate. Nausea and vomiting may also occur. Hemorrhoids will often become engorged. Fecal incontinence, with liquid stool leaking about the impaction, is common. An impaction may cause pressure on the bladder neck, obstructing urinary flow, resulting in overflow incontinence.

56. C: There are four classifications of neuropathic pain:

- Mononeuropathy: Involves only one nerve, such as with trigeminal neuralgia and herpes zoster.
- Polyneuropathy: Involves multiple nerves, such as with AIDS-associated, diabetic, and alcoholic neuropathy.
- Deafferentation: Input into the CNS is impaired, such as with post-herpetic syndrome and phantom pain associated with amputations.
- Sympathetically-mediated: Involves damage to the sympathetic nervous system, such as with complex regional pain syndrome.

57. A: Visceral pain frequently requires opioids to control although in early stages of disease when pain is less severe, patients may respond to NSAIDs. Neuropathic pain often responds poorly to opioids and is better treated with antidepressants, anticonvulsants, and/or benzodiazepines. Somatic pain may be treated with various drugs, including steroids, NSAIDs, muscle relaxants, and bisphosphonates. Psychological pain is usually treated with psychiatric treatment that may or may not include the use of psychotropic drugs.

58. D: If a patient has been self-medicating with 2000 mg of acetaminophen every 3 to 4 hours around the clock for back pain, believing it to be free of adverse effects, but the patient has developed acetaminophen toxicity, the recommended reversal agent is N-acetylcysteine. Serum levels of acetaminophen greater than 150 require the antidote N-acetylcysteine: 72-hour protocol begins with 140 mg/kg and 70 mg/kg every 4 hours for 17 more doses (administered orally or intravenously). Ideally, the antidote should be administered within 8 hours because of the risk of liver failure.

59. B: Because the patient is able to keep a record of pain medications, the patient is probably not confused or giving the medication to someone else. However, patients are often reluctant to admit the degree of pain and minimize their discomfort when asked about their pain, so it's important to determine how much pain medication the patient is actually taking and to observe the patient's behavior for indications of pain. Some patients may believe that having pain indicates their condition is poor and persist in saying they have little pain despite obvious evidence otherwise.

60. B: FACES (Wong-Baker): Facial expression scale used for children over 7. An adult version is also available. CHEOPS is used for children 1-7 and based on scores of 6 different characteristics (crying, facial expression, verbalization, torso, upper extremities, lower extremities). CRIES: Assesses crying, requirement for O2 or SaO2 <95%, increased VS, expression, and sleep to evaluate pain in neonates and infants 6 months or younger. The 0-10 pain intensity scale is used with adolescents and adults.

61. D: Naloxone is a reversal agent (opiate antagonist) used for opioids, such as morphine. Patients must be monitored for hypertension and pulmonary edema after administration, and since the half-life is only approximately 20 minutes, repeat doses may be needed. Flumazenil is a reversal agent for benzodiazepines. N-acetylcysteine is a reversal agent for acetaminophen. Neostigmine is a reversal agent for non-depolarizing muscle relaxants. Reversal agents should always be available when patients are receiving high doses of opioids or benzodiazepines.

62. C: Examples of Schedule IV drugs include benzodiazepines, tramadol, long acting barbiturates, butorphanol, pentazocine, and some antidiarrheal drugs (difenoxin). Schedule IV drugs have lower potential for abuse than drugs in Schedules I (illicit drugs), II (opioids), and III (anabolic steroids, intermediate acting barbiturates, and compounds with NSAIDS). Schedule IV drugs may still lead to limited physical and psychological dependence. For example, tramadol (which is widely prescribed) has been associated with overdoses.

63. D: Corticosteroids, such as prednisone or dexamethasone, are used as adjuvant analgesics to relieve pain associated with spinal cord compression, cerebral edema, and bone pain as well as visceral and neuropathic pain. Corticosteroids have anti-inflammatory effects that reduce swelling and inflammation. Prednisone may be given in doses of 15 to 30 mg three to four times daily. Dexamethasone is less likely to result in Cushing's syndrome than prednisone. Dexamethasone may be given orally at 2 to 20 mg a day or IV (up to 100 mg bolus) for severe pain crisis.

64. A: Eutectic Mixture of Local Anesthetics (EMLA Cream) provides good pain control. The skin is first cleansed and then the cream is applied thickly (1/4 inch) extending about 1/2 inch past the port to the peri-port tissue. The cream is then covered with plastic wrap, which is secured and left in place for about 20 minutes. The wrapped time may be extended to 45-60 minute if necessary, to completely numb the tissue. The tissue should remain numb for about 1 hour after the plastic wrap is removed, allowing time for the IV needle to be inserted and treatment begun.

65. C: <u>Physical dependence:</u> Abrupt cessation of a drug and decrease in blood serum levels leads to withdrawal symptoms, which may vary depending on the type of drug. <u>Addiction</u> is a neurobiological disorder that includes lack of control over drug use, compulsive use of drugs, and continued craving for drugs despite negative effects. <u>Tolerance</u> is an adaptation in which a drug's effect diminishes over time so that an increased dose is needed to achieve the same effect. <u>Pseudoaddiction</u> is the mistaken belief that someone who is seeking drugs for pain is instead suffering from addiction.

66. B: Morphine 10mg is equianalgesic to 1.5 mg of hydromorphone. Hydromorphone (Dilaudid®) is a hydrogenated ketone derivative of morphine. It is more highly lipid soluble than morphine and crosses the blood-brain barrier more readily, so it is faster acting than morphine and stronger (about 8 times). It has potent antitussive qualities. It produces less histamine release, nausea, and vomiting than morphine, so it is a good alternative if patients have an allergic response to morphine.

67. A: Asian cultures tend to value stoicism, so Asian patients may not express pain with moaning or complaints, so the pain management nurse cannot always use behavior as a guide when assessing a patient's degree of pain. Northern Europeans also tend to be fairly stoic. Hispanic, Middle Eastern, and southern European/Mediterranean cultures tend to be more expressive and their behavior may indicate pain is more severe than it actually is. While generalizations about culture may hold true for a culture as a whole, it's important to remember that they cannot necessarily be applied to any one individual in that culture.

68. A: This type of breakthrough pain is end-of-dose failure because the medication has peaked and the blood level is decreasing. A pain diary can help to establish the pattern of end-of-dose failure. The best solution is to either increase the dosage, usually by 25% to 50%, or to change the patch more frequently, such as every 48 hours. Increasing the use of oral opioids for the last 24 hours is not a good solution because the patient's pain is not being adequately controlled.

69. D: Most opioids can cause pruritus, but morphine, which causes more histamine release, is more likely to cause pruritus than other opioids such as fentanyl, codeine, and oxymorphone. If itching is mild, an antihistamine given concurrently may control itching, but in some cases discontinuing the morphine and switching to another drug or rotating between morphine and another drug may be necessary. Application of cold may help relieve itching to a localized area, but heat often increases itching. Topical anti-pruritics, such as hydrocortisone, may relieve itching but are not practical if itching is generalized.

70. C: The federal law that gives patients the right to make decisions about care based on informed consent and to accept or refuse treatment is the *Patient Self Determination Act* (1991). Patients must be informed of their rights and asked if they have advance directives. If so, a copy should be obtained and placed in the medical record. Patients who are of sound mind may refuse any treatment although the courts may, in rare cases, intervene in treatment decisions for minor children.

71. A: Patients with history of drug abuse are entitled to adequate pain control, but they must be assessed and evaluated carefully. Of special concern are patients who roll and smoke fentanyl patches because smoking the patch can release a 3-day supply of the drug rapidly and result in a life-threatening overdose. Patients with a history of drug abuse may have developed a tolerance to drugs, so taking medications before scheduled time and asking for higher doses are not uncommon although some patients react in the opposite way and are fearful of taking pain medications.

72. B: The Agency for Healthcare Policy and Research recommends use of the ABCDE method for assessing and managing pain:

    A. <u>Asking</u> patient about the extent of pain and assessing systematically.
    B. <u>Believing</u> that the degree of pain the patient reports is accurate.
    C. <u>Choosing</u> the appropriate method of pain control for the patient and circumstances.
    D. <u>Delivering</u> pain interventions appropriately and in a timely, logical manner.
    E. <u>Empowering</u> patients and family by helping them to have control of the course of treatment.

73. B: NSAIDS are contraindicated as co-adjuvants with corticosteroids because they have similar side effects and can increase the risk of gastrointestinal irritation and bleeding. NSAIDs may be used as sole analgesia initially to treat mild to moderate pain and are used as adjuvant drugs with opioids at steps 2 or 3 of the analgesic ladder. NSAIDs provide an antiinflammatory effect and are especially effective for reducing bone pain. While NSAIDS do not produce dependence or addiction and may reduce the need for opioids, they are associated with many adverse effects.

74. C: <u>Conditional</u> risk factors for substance abuse include health conditions, such as chronic disability and pain, mental health disorders (bipolar, schizophrenia, post-traumatic stress syndrome) and mood disorders (anxiety, depression). Other risk factors include <u>familial</u> (unstable home environment, abuse, person or familial history of substance abuse), <u>social</u> (association with members of gangs, low income, homelessness, low sense of self-esteem, low grades in school), and <u>professional</u> (healthcare workers with easy access to controlled substances coupled with emotional problems or stress).

75. D: <u>Bisphosphonates</u> are used specifically as adjuvant drugs to relieve osteolytic bone pain. <u>Tricyclic antidepressants</u> are used for burning neuropathic pain and to relieve insomnia or depression. Anticonvulsants are used for sharp, shooting, shock-like neuropathic pain. Corticosteroids have broad use for bone pain, neuropathic pain, visceral pain, and cord compression as well as pain crisis. Additionally, antispasmodics are used to reduce muscle spasms. Calcium channel blockers may reduce both ischemic and neuropathic pain and reduce smooth muscle spasms.

76. D: When a medication has provided good pain control but significant side effects occur, the dose of the new opioid should start at 25 to 50% below the equianalgesic dose in the event that cross-tolerant symptoms occur. Rescue doses may be given with breakthrough of pain. If, on the other hand, pain control was not adequate and significant side effects occurred, then opioids should be rotated at the equianalgesic dose. In either case, the patient must be monitored carefully for adverse effects.

77. A: If the starting dose proves ineffective and the patient requires more than 4 rescue doses in 24 hours, then the best action is to increase the baseline opioid dose. During titration, the dosage should be increased until optimal pain relief is achieved. Additionally, the rescue dosage should be increased along with the baseline dose so that they remain proportional. Generally, if one or two side effects occur, the medication is continued and side effects treated unless the side effects are severe. If more than two side effects occur, then opioid rotation may be indicated.

78. C: Distraction is most effective for short periods of discomfort, such as those associated with medical procedures, but it is less effective for severe acute pain or chronic pain although distraction may improve mood and relieve anxiety. Children are often distracted with toys, books, or games during procedures. Patient's interests should always be considered as distracting someone with something to which the person has no interest is not effective. Distraction may be primarily passive, as in watching television, or active, as in singing along with music or clapping hands.

79. D: A prolonged QTc of greater than 450 ms indicates that a patient considered for methadone treatment may be at increased risk of ventricular tachycardia or cardiac arrest with the drug. Therefore, the American Pain Society recommends that any patient at risk of ventricular tachycardia (history of previous prolongation to >450 or previous VT) should have an ECG before treatment with methadone is initiated. The APS also recommends that an ECG should be considered even if no risk factors are present.

80. C: Patients with constant severe pain should routinely receive pain medications around the clock. The frequency of administration depends on the degree of pain and the type of medication. The point of pain management is to avoid breakthrough pain, which can be debilitating and increase anxiety. Patients who are fearful of breakthrough pain may experience more pain because of anxiety. An important part of pain management is to anticipate adverse effects, such as constipation or sedation, and provide prophylaxis.

81. B: If a patient with an implanted pacemaker has persistent low-back pain and asks the pain management nurse about using a TENS machine that a friend loaned the patient, the pain management nurse should advise the patient that a TENS machine is contraindicated with a pacemaker because it may interfere with the pacemaker functioning. The patient should also be advised to avoid using other people's medical equipment or taking other people's medications.

82. D: The patient's inability to understand oral instructions and disinterest in illustrations suggests a kinesthetic learner, so the nurse should allow the patient to handle the equipment and practice. Kinesthetic learns learn best by handling, doing, and practicing with minimal directions and hands-on experience. Other learning styles include:

Visual learners learn best by seeing and reading:

- Provide written directions, picture guides, or demonstrate procedures.
- Use charts and diagrams.
- Provide photos, videos.

Auditory learners learn best by listening and talking:

- Explain procedures while demonstrating and have learner repeat.
- Plan extra time to discuss and answer questions.
- Provide audiotapes.

83. B: When doing a heel prick or blood draw on a young infant, the best pain relief is likely derived from having the infant suck on a pacifier dipped in 24% sucrose solution. The sucrose is believed to act in the brain in a manner similar to opioids. While non-nutritive sucking alone can provide some comfort for the infant, the addition of sucrose provides better control of pain. The child should be given the pacifier 1 to 2 minutes prior to the procedure. Analgesia last 3-5 minutes.

84. B: To effectively use guided imagery and visualization as a relaxation technique to reduce anxiety and pain, the child should generally be over 6 years old. Younger children usually have difficulty focusing the attention for a prolonged period. To teach the child, the nurse management nurse should ask the child to imagine a favorite place, such as a park or Disneyland, and try to image the sights, sounds, smells, touches, and feelings and to think about what it's like to be there.

85. C: Soaking dressing to loosen prior to removal relieves cyclic acute pain. CWPE model:

- Non-cyclic acute wound pain: Occurs with trauma, such as sharp debridement. Interventions include topical or local anesthetics and anti-anxiety medication.
- Cyclic acute wound pain: Occurs at regular times, such as with wound changes or position changes. Interventions include soaking dressing, timeouts, non-adherent dressings, and use of repositioning devices.
- Chronic wound pain: Occurs continuously. Interventions include heat, transcutaneous nerve stimulation, and tricyclic antidepressants.

86. D: If a patient with bone cancer has been reluctant to take adequate analgesia because it conflicts with his self-image as a stoic, strong, active man, but the pain restricts his functional abilities, leading to depression and anxiety, the best approach for the pain management nurse is to focus on how pain medication can increase functional abilities. The patient's need to appear strong and active has served as a barrier to pain management, so focusing on how pain medication can help maintain what is important to him is essential.

87. A: Three to 5 minutes. Procedure for lidocaine soak:

1. Draw 5 to 10 mL of 2% lidocaine into a syringe.
2. Remove wound dressing and cleanse wound.
3. Place clean dry gauze over surface of wound.
4. Saturate the wound area (and gauze) with the 2% lidocaine.
5. Allow the lidocaine solution to contact the wound for 3 to 5 minutes.
6. Evaluate pain sensation to ensure the area is anesthetized.
7. Debride wound and redress as appropriate.

88. B: If morphine is administered subcutaneously, peak analgesia occurs in 20 minutes. With the oral route, peak analgesia occurs in 60 minutes; with intramuscular, 30 to 60 minutes; with intravenous, 20 minutes; and rectally, 20 to 60 minutes. Morphine is much less potent ($1/3^{rd}$ to $1/6^{th}$) orally compared to intravenous administration because oral bioavailability of the drug ranges from 20% to 40%.

89. A: If a patient has second-degree burns on both hands with blistering and sloughing of outer layers of skin, the patient is likely experiencing severe pain. Initial treatment to control pain from burns generally includes an IV opioid, such as 0.1 mg/kg morphine sulfate (in titrated boluses until pain controlled). An alternative is 1.5mcg/kg intranasal fentanyl, which is also rapid acting. Once the patient's pain level is stabilized, the patient may switch to oral analgesia.

90. C: "What causes the pain?"

PQRST Method of pain assessment		
P	Perception/Provoking factors	What causes the pain? What relieves the pain or makes it worse?
Q	Quality of pain	What does the pain feel like? Would you describe the pain as sharp, dull, stabbing, shock-like, aching, burning?
R	Radiation	Does the pain move or stay in one place?
S	Severity	Can you rank the pain on a scale of 1 to 10?
T	Time (onset and duration)	When did the pain start? How long did it last?

91. A: One of the best positions to relieve acute back pain is side-lying curled position with knees and hips flexed and a pillow separating knees although patients should be encouraged to change position and alternate periods of sitting, standing, and lying. Positions that increase lordosis, such as the prone position, may increase pain for many people. Sitting should be done in a firm chair with arm support and pillow at back to facilitate standing. Some people find that lying on a firm surface with head elevated to 30° and knees slightly elevated also reduces discomfort.

92. D: If in reviewing a patient's records, the pain management nurse notes that the patient's pain seems poorly controlled when under the care of one particular nurse, but that nurse has documented that the patient receives the medication every 4 hours as prescribed, the pain management nurse should suspect that the nurse is diverting the patient's medications. One method of diversion is to replace opioid tablets with acetaminophen or an NSAID and to replace an injectable drug with NS or sterile water.

93. B: When applying an ice pack to a patient's lower back (or any other body part) to relieve pain, the maximum duration of time the ice pack should be left in place each time is 20 minutes, and the ice pack should be covered with a cloth so that the pack does not lie directly against the skin.

Treatment with ice packs may be repeated 8 to 10 times a day. Ice packs are contraindicated in areas with poor perfusion or impaired sensation.

94. C: The primary treatment for moderate to severe cancer-related pain is opioids, such as morphine or fentanyl. Moderate to severe pain is usually associated with metastatic or advanced cancer, so the concern is to keep the patient as comfortable as possible at the end of life with less concern about the potential for addiction although patients may develop tolerance to drugs and require increasing dosages or different drugs in order to maintain comfort levels. Even with opioids, some cancer-related pain may be difficult to control.

95. A: According to the Pain Care Bill of Rights, patients have the right to:

- Have pain thoroughly assessed and treated.
- Be treated with dignity and respect when reporting pain.
- Be advised of causes, potential treatments, risks and benefits, and costs.
- Be an active participant in decision-making.
- Undergo periodic reassessment and modification of treatment.
- Receive a referral to a pain specialist if needed.
- Receive answers to questions and refuse treatments.

96. C: If a patient with Guillain-Barré syndrome reports severe pain but the patient's facial expression has remained unchanged, this probably indicates flaccid facial paralysis, a common finding. Patients with GBS often complain of severe burning pain in affected muscles. Pain may be an early symptom, often occurring before the onset of weakness and paralysis. Treatment options include NSAIDs, opioids, anticonvulsants, and tricyclic antidepressants.

97. D: The cause of post mastectomy pain syndrome is direct damage to the nerves. The pain may be severe and intractable causing much distress and impairing the patient's ability to function. Pain is typical of neuropathic pain—burning, tingling, numbness—and may include a feeling of muscle constriction. Various methods of pain control include the use of tricyclic antidepressants, anticonvulsants, capsaicin, and fat grafting (a surgical procedure).

98. B: When using diclofenac sodium 1% gel for relief of joint pain, the patient should ensure the right dosage by using the plastic dosing card/ruler that comes with the tube of medicine. The gel can be applied directly onto the card to the correct dosage (2 g equal 2.25 inches; 4 g equal 4.5 inches) and then wiped off with a finger and applied to the joint. The card should be rinsed clean between applications.

99. A: The Gate Control Theory of Pain explains why pain is sometimes blocked and other times not. According to this theory, pain signals travel through a number of "gates," and the more gates that are open, the greater the perception of pain. Cognitive, sensory, and psychological influences may all affect whether gates are opened or closed. For example, stress and injury may open gates while relaxation and positive thoughts may close gates and lesson the perception of pain.

100. C: Since treatments should begin with the least invasive, the mirror box should be tried next to relieve phantom pain. The patient inserts his intact arm into one side of the box and his stump into the other side of the box. The box is separated by a center mirror. The patient then moves the intact arm and hand and observes the image reflected in the mirror, imagining that the image is his amputated limb. This "tricks" the brain into thinking the arm is intact and relieves pain in a significant number of people.

101. C: Nociception refers to programming and recognizing deleterious (noxious) stimuli when it transmits to a sensory receptor (nociceptor). The stimulus and reaction of the nociceptors result in the sensation of pain that is known as nociceptive pain. Nociceptive pain subtypes include visceral pain (from the organs or the lining of the organs), often characterized by cramping, and somatic pain (skin, subcutaneous layers, bones, muscles, and blood vessels) frequently described as specific to a localized area, throbbing, stabbing, or aching. Nociceptors respond in distinctive ways to severe thermal, chemical, and mechanical stimuli. Neuropathic pain (pathological) originates in the peripheral or central nervous system and may be prolonged by unusual somatosensory processing in these systems. The subtypes of neuropathic pain include "central generator," which is deafferentation, central, or phantom pain, or sympathetic pain. The second type is "peripheral generator," which begins in the nerve root, plexus, or nerve.

102. B: Melzack promoted the Neuromatrix Model of Pain, which maintains that pain develops from complicated neuromatrices consisting of parallel and redundant neurological and neurochemical systems inside the brain, which are not bound by activity in an isolated sensory cortex. Information received from the various systems combines in the brain to produce the pain experience. The specificity theory hypothesizes that pain is not a punishment for misdeeds, as believed in ancient times, or an emotion, as postulated by Aristotle, but related to specific anatomical and physiological functions. Melzack and Wall's gate control theory states that pain is a multifaceted perceptual experience that evolves from that individual's exclusive psychological and physiological factors. The pattern theory evolved to explain unique examples of pain such as phantom limb sensation, allodynia, or hyperalgesia.

103. C: Fibromyalgia syndrome refers to chronic mild to severe soft-tissue pain and allodynia. Symptoms include continuous pain, which may vary in intensity, interrupting sleep patterns. Central sensitization results in a magnified awareness of pain. Chronic exhaustion plus muscle and joint stiffness near the maximum range of motion frequently accompany this condition. Temporomandibular joint dysfunction is a frequent cause of orofacial pain. Radiculopathy refers to a spinal nerve root disorder. Peripheral neuropathy is associated with injury to a specific peripheral nerve.

104. A: The education of health-care professionals on the latest recommended guidelines for cancer pain management results in optimal pain management. Opioid therapy is more than 75% effective in treating cancer pain. NSAIDs, administered orally, are effective in certain cancer pain syndromes. Subcutaneous infusion of opioids is a cost savings for the patient because it does not demand the skill level of other routes of administration.

105. A: Hyperalgesia is an exaggerated or amplified response to painful stimuli, which may manifest itself in various ways, most likely due to the cause of the peripheral stimulus. Neuropathic pain sufferers frequently complain of cutaneous hypersensitivity and amplified pain due to mechanical and thermal stimuli. Windup is a progressive increase in the scale of response to C fiber activity. Long-term potentiation is the concept that a cellular memory for pain may lead to future increased responses to nociceptive stimuli. The development of a situation in which, due to recurring excitement of a neuron, the impulse threshold decreases and the strength of the response increases is called facilitation.

106. C: Neuromas frequently form after limb amputation. They form on damaged myelinated and unmyelinated nerve fibers, and they may be tiny and difficult to palpate. If a neuroma is located inside scar tissue, ongoing stimulation may occur, causing a condition that is referred to as neuromas in continuity.

107. D: Caring implies a commitment to all the bioethical principles (Thompson, 1996). Caring is a willingness to respect the patient's informed choices based on his or her values and beliefs.

108. C: Unresolved pain and the ensuing stress hormone release may cause several negative physical effects, including increased myocardial oxygen consumption, tachycardia, hypercoagulability (leading to increase in deep vein thrombosis), immunosuppression, and unrelenting catabolism. Pain also decreases gastric motility.

109. A: The definition of breach of duty is the failure of the pain management nurse to provide reasonable care. Examples include the failure to observe and report an infection at the site of an epidural injection. Opioid administration is part of the pain management nurse's job. The staff must have ongoing appropriate pain management education. Failure to report significant changes in the patient's condition is a breach of duty.

110. A: The determination of the intensity of acute pain may be accomplished by the use of existing tools. These include the Visual Analog Scale (VAS) and the Numeric Pain Intensity Scale. The McGill Pain Questionnaire measures experimentally induced and postprocedural pain. The Pain Outcomes Questionnaire is used to assess chronic pain. The Brief Pain Inventory (BPI) was developed for patients with cancer pain and is now used in the assessment of other types of chronic pain.

111. B: Included in the Checklist of Nonverbal Pain Indicators (CNPI) are activities that include facial grimacing, rubbing, bracing, restlessness, vocalizations, and vocal complaints. Staring into space and sleeping are usually signs of relaxation.

112. D: The objective of the acute pain assessment tools is to evaluate the pain so that relief or reduction of pain may be achieved. Tools should be easy to use, quick, and simple, providing documentable data for assessment and reassessment. These tools need to be understandable by patients of all languages and cultures. They are necessary for rapid evaluation. More comprehensive, complex testing may be required as treatment progresses, but the first objective is to quickly evaluate and relieve the acute pain.

113. C: "Feels very sad," describes the way the face "feels" instead of the pain level. Use words like "hurt" or "pain" to describe the faces, not "sad" or "happy," which describe emotion.

114. D: Studies have shown that all individuals, regardless of background, have similar neurophysiological systems of pain perception. Minorities may be at greater risk for inadequate pain treatment, but the pain management nurse must avoid prejudging based on cultural or ethnic heritage. Some cultures have firm beliefs regarding the expression of pain, so observation for nonverbal signs is important.

115. C: The repetition of the patient's statements in an attempt to elicit more details regarding the pain they are experiencing is a technique called reflection. Actions such as touching the patient's arm, leaning forward in your chair, and maintaining eye contact and words of encouragement are all examples of facilitation. Statements that indicate empathy and understanding fall under the heading of empathetic response. Asking for an explanation of what a patient means by a statement or by unusual behavior is an example of clarification.

116. C: Patients with dementia may not be able to accurately self-report pain. Mentally competent patients with rheumatic disease, chronic pain, or cancer pain would be able to use the Numeric Pain Intensity Scale.

117. B: Asking about what makes the pain better would be an attempt to determine the alleviating or relieving factor. Constipation, nausea, vomiting, and lack of sleep due to the pain are associative factors.

118. B: The use of the FACES Scale in pediatric patients is a legitimate means of determining pain level. The Verbal Descriptive Scale (VDS), Brief Pain Inventory (BPI), and the McGill Pain Inventory are too complex for the typical pediatric patient.

119. B: The Verbal Descriptor Scale (VDS) is a <u>uni</u>dimensional assessment tool, which uses verbal descriptors such as no pain, mild pain, moderate pain, severe pain, very severe pain, and worst pain possible. Examples of multidimensional pain scales are the McGill Pain Questionnaire, the Brief Pain Inventory (BPI), the West Haven-Yale Multidimensional Pain Inventory, and the Pain Outcomes Questionnaire. Multidimensional pain scales assess more than just intensity, nature, and location, they also evaluate mood, drug efficacy, and the effect the pain is having on the patient's daily life and sleep patterns.

120. A: The Opioid Risk Tool (ORT) contains a brief list of questions including any family history or personal history of substance abuse, age, preadolescent sexual abuse, psychological disease, or depression. Psoriasis, hypertension, high cholesterol, diabetes, and heart disease would be concerns, but they would not be significant to the ORT.

121. C: Lack of adequate pain management education, misconceptions regarding medications, addictions and pain, and attitudinal concerns combine to prevent proper pain alleviation. In the U.S., there is an ample supply of pain medications.

122. D: Poorly controlled pain hastens death due to the increased psychological stress, diminished immunocompetence, reduced mobility, higher incidence of pneumonia and thromboembolism, and increased oxygen requirements.

123. C: Acetaminophen has a limited anti-inflammatory action. It does work well as a "coanalgesic" for severe pain and for nonspecific musculoskeletal pain. Its usage should be limited in patients that use significant amounts of alcohol or have liver or kidney disease.

124. A: Nonsteroidal anti-inflammatory drugs (NSAIDs) reduce biosynthesis of prostaglandins, which decreases the cascade of inflammatory episodes that cause, maintain, or increase nociception. Their secondary mode of analgesic effectiveness is not completely understood. Opioids are nonspecific and decrease the pain signal throughout the nervous system. Fentanyl is available in several different modes of administration, including patch and transmucosal means. The side effects of morphine are constipation, itching, headache, dysphoria, sedation, and nausea.

125. C: Addiction is a primary, chronic, neurobiological disease characterized by compulsive cravings for a drug, lack of control over its usage, and continued use even when harmful effects have occurred. Tolerance is a state of adaptation in which exposure to a drug produces changes that result in minimal effectiveness of one or more of the drug's usual actions. Physical dependence is a state of adaptation that results in a withdrawal syndrome that can be elicited by a sudden dose reduction or cessation. Pseudotolerance is the misconception that the necessity of increasing the dosage of a drug is due to tolerance instead of an increase in the severity of pain.

126. A: Clearance is the amount of blood that is totally free of the medication in a set period. Elimination refers to the process that takes place that results in the excretion of drugs through the kidneys. Enzyme induction is an adaptive reaction, which protects cells by augmenting the function of the liver enzymes, thus decreasing the extent of the drug's effect. Biotransformation is the process by which drugs are broken down to water-soluble compounds, or metabolites.

127. D: Pharmacodynamics is the reaction of tissue to certain chemical agents at different locations in the body. Mechanism of action refers to the change in function at the site of action resulting from the absorption of the drug. Cmax is the term that indicates the maximum concentration of the drug, also known as the peak level. Efficacy is the capability of a drug to instigate biological activity in the drug-receptor interaction.

128. C: A patient with a history of prolonged opioid usage who complains of constipation is experiencing a side effect, which is a predictable reaction that has been frequently observed in the population and is expected. Overdose or toxicity results from an excessive drug level in the blood. An allergic reaction can be anaphylactic and involves an immune response. A drug interaction is a modification of the degree or duration of the action of one drug when used in conjunction with another drug.

129. A: The technique of using NSAIDs, COX-2 inhibitors (coxib), or acetaminophen in combination with an opioid for effective pain management is multimodal analgesia. Therapeutic drug monitoring refers to monitoring blood plasma levels of a drug. Pharmacokinetics refers to the process by which a drug moves to the target site, is detoxified, and is eliminated from the body. Genetic polymorphism is the number of people within a population who will inherit liver enzyme activity that is controlled by a single genetic locus.

130. B: Antagonists produce the reversal of analgesia, recovery from respiratory depression, relief of opioid-induced constipation, and treatment of opioid withdrawal. Steroids (glucocorticoid steroid) produce anti-inflammatory actions. Hypnotics are used for the short-term treatment of insomnia. Anxiolytic drugs are effective in reducing anxiety and for their anticonvulsant and antispasmodic effects.

131. A: Preemptive analgesia prevents the establishment of altered central processing of afferent input. The administration of analgesic drugs prior to a procedure or surgery (nociceptive event) decreases the occurrence of hyperalgesia and allodynia. Multimodal analgesia refers to a combination of medications that work on different sites in the peripheral and central nervous systems. An agent that blocks or removes a sensation is an anesthetic. Agonists are drugs that bind to physiological receptors and imitate the effects of endogenous signaling compounds.

132. B: PCA does not refer to the delivery pump, but to the method of analgesia therapy.

133. C: The main disadvantage of the bolus dose with PCA is that the patient must be awake to administer the medication.

134. D: Constipation often accompanies opioid usage. The administration of stool softeners may be indicated as a precaution. Itching, urinary retention, respiratory depression, nausea and vomiting, and sedation are serious side effects associated with continuous administration. The nursing assessment includes respiratory status, including the various characteristics of the respirations, signs of oversedation, and frequent monitoring for side effects.

135. C: Preventive measures for reducing the occurrence of chronic pain include various lifestyle changes. Maintaining an ideal weight minimizes pain associated with the lower back, joint disease, and diabetes. Exercise improves circulation, averts muscle atrophy, increases muscle tone, and helps prevent osteoporosis. Correct posture and lifting techniques decrease the occurrence of back, shoulder, and neck pain. The cessation of smoking decreases back pain and peripheral circulation disease. Minimal alcohol consumption lowers the incidence of alcohol neuropathy and pancreatitis. Decreasing stress levels improves sleep patterns, healing, and the patient's ability to deal with pain. Heat therapy, hydrotherapy and biofeedback are not preventative measures of pain, but rather can be used to help ease already occurring pain.

136. A: The goals for patient education regarding pain include decreasing their misunderstandings regarding pain, increasing their observance of pain regimens, emphasizing family-centered care, facilitating communication between the care provider and the patient, improving pain relief, increasing the patient's knowledge and awareness, and developing the patient's skills related to their pain control methods. Improving the patient's understanding of medical jargon is inappropriate; communication needs to be clear and understandable. The patient should be encouraged to talk with others about their pain.

137. D: Adults with a low literacy level require a different approach to education. Low literacy does not equate with low intelligence; it simply means the patient may not have the ability to read, comprehend, or use written information effectively. The patient educator should use simple sentences and visual cues to express essential information. Emphasis should be placed on important content by beginning and ending with it. The reading levels of educational materials need to be assessed by the educator. The patient needs to be involved in the class and be encouraged to ask questions; therefore, lectures are not the ideal presentation technique.

138. A: The best tools for evaluation of the patient's comprehension include testing and retesting, return demonstrations, repetition of content, surveys, and the patient's written evaluation of the class content, presentation, and atmosphere. Although the educator's background can play a role in the style of presentation, if the material is covered properly, this should not be a factor. The patient's level of participation in group discussions may indicate a lack of confidence in a group setting, a fear of public speaking or ridicule, or other personal concerns.

139. D: Cancer patient education should include several concepts: most pain can be relieved, there is no advantage to enduring pain, patients need to learn to describe and measure pain levels, pain can often be mitigated by a multimodal approach, options other than medication are available, morphine and similar drugs are frequently used, and medications for pain should be stored in a safe place. Other suggestions consist of stressing clear communication between the patient and professional staff, the patient's knowledge of the medication's names, when to take the drug, possible side effects and how to deal with them, noninvasive therapies, and contact information or help. Follow-up is important, and the plan should be made clear.

140. B: Testing and retesting are excellent tools for evaluating the patient's comprehension of the material. Common errors made by teachers include an incomplete needs assessment, using information that is too complex, and not getting feedback to evaluate the patient's comprehension of the presented materials.

141. B: The educator's best approach is to meet with the patient in private and assess their motivation and readiness level. The educator should not stop the class when other patients are involved. Setting goals and objectives is an important step in educating the patient, but this step comes after ascertaining motivation and readiness levels. Documentation of pertinent information obtained during the session is part of the education process.

142. D: The goals of public education on pain management include an increased awareness and knowledge of pain management in the community, a decrease in misconceptions regarding pain treatment, and assistance in facilitating access to suitable health care. Assessing individual needs of audience members is not a primary goal of public education.

143. A: This statement is an example of myths and misconceptions. Literacy is the ability to read, understand, and utilize the information. Socioeconomic status and education level should be assessed, but this statement reflects a myth or misconception about pain management.

144. D: The patient who has literacy deficiencies is less likely to follow instructions, may fail to seek preventative care, and may have difficulty understanding how to use the health-care system. This patient is more likely to make medication errors and misunderstand medication labels. If the patient is using the medication properly, their pain relief should be adequate.

145. D: Documentation of the educational session should include the content provided in the session, the outcomes of the education (if the patient can demonstrate the skill), and the next step in the education plan. Patients' spiritual beliefs are not included in this documentation.

146. B: The didactic method of teaching includes lecturing with the addition of slides, videos, teleconference, handouts, and Web-based education. Clinical practicum refers to an interactive training program for nurses. Andragogy is the term used for the art and science of teaching adults, and pedagogy is the term for the art and science of teaching children.

147. D: The standards of practice for the pain management nurse require the nurse to be continually up to date, not just take courses every five years. Other standards include providing education for the patient and family, teaching ancillary personnel specific and appropriate aspects of pain management, and mentor and serve as a resource for nurses with limited pain management knowledge.

148. B: Mental illness, anxiety, grief, and cultural and language differences are all examples of patient and family barriers to education. Common errors in teaching refer to the inadequacy of the educator's techniques. Professional barriers and systemic barriers are problems with the providers of service.

149. C: The core curriculum for the pain management nurse does not include a course on prescriptive authority and prescription writing skills.

150. C: The transtheoretical model affirms that a deliberate change requires nonlinear movement through discrete motivational stages over time, with relapse and return to earlier stages before eventually succeeding. In the pain stages of change model, four distinct scales are used. The representational approach to patient education purports that individuals have thoughts about their health problem that include labels associated with the illness, beliefs about its origin, ideas about the timeline, consequences, and convictions about the possibilities of a cure.

How to Overcome Test Anxiety

Just the thought of taking a test is enough to make most people a little nervous. A test is an important event that can have a long-term impact on your future, so it's important to take it seriously and it's natural to feel anxious about performing well. But just because anxiety is normal, that doesn't mean that it's helpful in test taking, or that you should simply accept it as part of your life. Anxiety can have a variety of effects. These effects can be mild, like making you feel slightly nervous, or severe, like blocking your ability to focus or remember even a simple detail.

If you experience test anxiety—whether severe or mild—it's important to know how to beat it. To discover this, first you need to understand what causes test anxiety.

Causes of Test Anxiety

While we often think of anxiety as an uncontrollable emotional state, it can actually be caused by simple, practical things. One of the most common causes of test anxiety is that a person does not feel adequately prepared for their test. This feeling can be the result of many different issues such as poor study habits or lack of organization, but the most common culprit is time management. Starting to study too late, failing to organize your study time to cover all of the material, or being distracted while you study will mean that you're not well prepared for the test. This may lead to cramming the night before, which will cause you to be physically and mentally exhausted for the test. Poor time management also contributes to feelings of stress, fear, and hopelessness as you realize you are not well prepared but don't know what to do about it.

Other times, test anxiety is not related to your preparation for the test but comes from unresolved fear. This may be a past failure on a test, or poor performance on tests in general. It may come from comparing yourself to others who seem to be performing better or from the stress of living up to expectations. Anxiety may be driven by fears of the future—how failure on this test would affect your educational and career goals. These fears are often completely irrational, but they can still negatively impact your test performance.

Review Video: 3 Reasons You Have Test Anxiety
Visit mometrix.com/academy and enter code: 428468

Elements of Test Anxiety

As mentioned earlier, test anxiety is considered to be an emotional state, but it has physical and mental components as well. Sometimes you may not even realize that you are suffering from test anxiety until you notice the physical symptoms. These can include trembling hands, rapid heartbeat, sweating, nausea, and tense muscles. Extreme anxiety may lead to fainting or vomiting. Obviously, any of these symptoms can have a negative impact on testing. It is important to recognize them as soon as they begin to occur so that you can address the problem before it damages your performance.

> **Review Video: 3 Ways to Tell You Have Test Anxiety**
> Visit mometrix.com/academy and enter code: 927847

The mental components of test anxiety include trouble focusing and inability to remember learned information. During a test, your mind is on high alert, which can help you recall information and stay focused for an extended period of time. However, anxiety interferes with your mind's natural processes, causing you to blank out, even on the questions you know well. The strain of testing during anxiety makes it difficult to stay focused, especially on a test that may take several hours. Extreme anxiety can take a huge mental toll, making it difficult not only to recall test information but even to understand the test questions or pull your thoughts together.

> **Review Video: How Test Anxiety Affects Memory**
> Visit mometrix.com/academy and enter code: 609003

Effects of Test Anxiety

Test anxiety is like a disease—if left untreated, it will get progressively worse. Anxiety leads to poor performance, and this reinforces the feelings of fear and failure, which in turn lead to poor performances on subsequent tests. It can grow from a mild nervousness to a crippling condition. If allowed to progress, test anxiety can have a big impact on your schooling, and consequently on your future.

Test anxiety can spread to other parts of your life. Anxiety on tests can become anxiety in any stressful situation, and blanking on a test can turn into panicking in a job situation. But fortunately, you don't have to let anxiety rule your testing and determine your grades. There are a number of relatively simple steps you can take to move past anxiety and function normally on a test and in the rest of life.

> **Review Video: How Test Anxiety Impacts Your Grades**
> Visit mometrix.com/academy and enter code: 939819

Physical Steps for Beating Test Anxiety

While test anxiety is a serious problem, the good news is that it can be overcome. It doesn't have to control your ability to think and remember information. While it may take time, you can begin taking steps today to beat anxiety.

Just as your first hint that you may be struggling with anxiety comes from the physical symptoms, the first step to treating it is also physical. Rest is crucial for having a clear, strong mind. If you are tired, it is much easier to give in to anxiety. But if you establish good sleep habits, your body and mind will be ready to perform optimally, without the strain of exhaustion. Additionally, sleeping well helps you to retain information better, so you're more likely to recall the answers when you see the test questions.

Getting good sleep means more than going to bed on time. It's important to allow your brain time to relax. Take study breaks from time to time so it doesn't get overworked, and don't study right before bed. Take time to rest your mind before trying to rest your body, or you may find it difficult to fall asleep.

> **Review Video: The Importance of Sleep for Your Brain**
> Visit mometrix.com/academy and enter code: 319338

Along with sleep, other aspects of physical health are important in preparing for a test. Good nutrition is vital for good brain function. Sugary foods and drinks may give a burst of energy but this burst is followed by a crash, both physically and emotionally. Instead, fuel your body with protein and vitamin-rich foods.

Also, drink plenty of water. Dehydration can lead to headaches and exhaustion, especially if your brain is already under stress from the rigors of the test. Particularly if your test is a long one, drink water during the breaks. And if possible, take an energy-boosting snack to eat between sections.

> **Review Video: How Diet Can Affect your Mood**
> Visit mometrix.com/academy and enter code: 624317

Along with sleep and diet, a third important part of physical health is exercise. Maintaining a steady workout schedule is helpful, but even taking 5-minute study breaks to walk can help get your blood pumping faster and clear your head. Exercise also releases endorphins, which contribute to a positive feeling and can help combat test anxiety.

When you nurture your physical health, you are also contributing to your mental health. If your body is healthy, your mind is much more likely to be healthy as well. So take time to rest, nourish your body with healthy food and water, and get moving as much as possible. Taking these physical steps will make you stronger and more able to take the mental steps necessary to overcome test anxiety.

> **Review Video: How to Stay Healthy and Prevent Test Anxiety**
> Visit mometrix.com/academy and enter code: 877894

Mental Steps for Beating Test Anxiety

Working on the mental side of test anxiety can be more challenging, but as with the physical side, there are clear steps you can take to overcome it. As mentioned earlier, test anxiety often stems from lack of preparation, so the obvious solution is to prepare for the test. Effective studying may be the most important weapon you have for beating test anxiety, but you can and should employ several other mental tools to combat fear.

First, boost your confidence by reminding yourself of past success—tests or projects that you aced. If you're putting as much effort into preparing for this test as you did for those, there's no reason you should expect to fail here. Work hard to prepare; then trust your preparation.

Second, surround yourself with encouraging people. It can be helpful to find a study group, but be sure that the people you're around will encourage a positive attitude. If you spend time with others who are anxious or cynical, this will only contribute to your own anxiety. Look for others who are motivated to study hard from a desire to succeed, not from a fear of failure.

Third, reward yourself. A test is physically and mentally tiring, even without anxiety, and it can be helpful to have something to look forward to. Plan an activity following the test, regardless of the outcome, such as going to a movie or getting ice cream.

When you are taking the test, if you find yourself beginning to feel anxious, remind yourself that you know the material. Visualize successfully completing the test. Then take a few deep, relaxing breaths and return to it. Work through the questions carefully but with confidence, knowing that you are capable of succeeding.

Developing a healthy mental approach to test taking will also aid in other areas of life. Test anxiety affects more than just the actual test—it can be damaging to your mental health and even contribute to depression. It's important to beat test anxiety before it becomes a problem for more than testing.

Review Video: Test Anxiety and Depression
Visit mometrix.com/academy and enter code: 904704

Study Strategy

Being prepared for the test is necessary to combat anxiety, but what does being prepared look like? You may study for hours on end and still not feel prepared. What you need is a strategy for test prep. The next few pages outline our recommended steps to help you plan out and conquer the challenge of preparation.

STEP 1: SCOPE OUT THE TEST

Learn everything you can about the format (multiple choice, essay, etc.) and what will be on the test. Gather any study materials, course outlines, or sample exams that may be available. Not only will this help you to prepare, but knowing what to expect can help to alleviate test anxiety.

STEP 2: MAP OUT THE MATERIAL

Look through the textbook or study guide and make note of how many chapters or sections it has. Then divide these over the time you have. For example, if a book has 15 chapters and you have five days to study, you need to cover three chapters each day. Even better, if you have the time, leave an extra day at the end for overall review after you have gone through the material in depth.

If time is limited, you may need to prioritize the material. Look through it and make note of which sections you think you already have a good grasp on, and which need review. While you are studying, skim quickly through the familiar sections and take more time on the challenging parts. Write out your plan so you don't get lost as you go. Having a written plan also helps you feel more in control of the study, so anxiety is less likely to arise from feeling overwhelmed at the amount to cover.

STEP 3: GATHER YOUR TOOLS

Decide what study method works best for you. Do you prefer to highlight in the book as you study and then go back over the highlighted portions? Or do you type out notes of the important information? Or is it helpful to make flashcards that you can carry with you? Assemble the pens, index cards, highlighters, post-it notes, and any other materials you may need so you won't be distracted by getting up to find things while you study.

If you're having a hard time retaining the information or organizing your notes, experiment with different methods. For example, try color-coding by subject with colored pens, highlighters, or post-it notes. If you learn better by hearing, try recording yourself reading your notes so you can listen while in the car, working out, or simply sitting at your desk. Ask a friend to quiz you from your flashcards, or try teaching someone the material to solidify it in your mind.

STEP 4: CREATE YOUR ENVIRONMENT

It's important to avoid distractions while you study. This includes both the obvious distractions like visitors and the subtle distractions like an uncomfortable chair (or a too-comfortable couch that makes you want to fall asleep). Set up the best study environment possible: good lighting and a comfortable work area. If background music helps you focus, you may want to turn it on, but otherwise keep the room quiet. If you are using a computer to take notes, be sure you don't have any other windows open, especially applications like social media, games, or anything else that could distract you. Silence your phone and turn off notifications. Be sure to keep water close by so you stay hydrated while you study (but avoid unhealthy drinks and snacks).

Also, take into account the best time of day to study. Are you freshest first thing in the morning? Try to set aside some time then to work through the material. Is your mind clearer in the afternoon or evening? Schedule your study session then. Another method is to study at the same time of day that you will take the test, so that your brain gets used to working on the material at that time and will be ready to focus at test time.

STEP 5: STUDY!

Once you have done all the study preparation, it's time to settle into the actual studying. Sit down, take a few moments to settle your mind so you can focus, and begin to follow your study plan. Don't give in to distractions or let yourself procrastinate. This is your time to prepare so you'll be ready to fearlessly approach the test. Make the most of the time and stay focused.

Of course, you don't want to burn out. If you study too long you may find that you're not retaining the information very well. Take regular study breaks. For example, taking five minutes out of every hour to walk briskly, breathing deeply and swinging your arms, can help your mind stay fresh.

As you get to the end of each chapter or section, it's a good idea to do a quick review. Remind yourself of what you learned and work on any difficult parts. When you feel that you've mastered the material, move on to the next part. At the end of your study session, briefly skim through your notes again.

But while review is helpful, cramming last minute is NOT. If at all possible, work ahead so that you won't need to fit all your study into the last day. Cramming overloads your brain with more information than it can process and retain, and your tired mind may struggle to recall even previously learned information when it is overwhelmed with last-minute study. Also, the urgent nature of cramming and the stress placed on your brain contribute to anxiety. You'll be more likely to go to the test feeling unprepared and having trouble thinking clearly.

So don't cram, and don't stay up late before the test, even just to review your notes at a leisurely pace. Your brain needs rest more than it needs to go over the information again. In fact, plan to finish your studies by noon or early afternoon the day before the test. Give your brain the rest of the day to relax or focus on other things, and get a good night's sleep. Then you will be fresh for the test and better able to recall what you've studied.

STEP 6: TAKE A PRACTICE TEST

Many courses offer sample tests, either online or in the study materials. This is an excellent resource to check whether you have mastered the material, as well as to prepare for the test format and environment.

Check the test format ahead of time: the number of questions, the type (multiple choice, free response, etc.), and the time limit. Then create a plan for working through them. For example, if you have 30 minutes to take a 60-question test, your limit is 30 seconds per question. Spend less time on the questions you know well so that you can take more time on the difficult ones.

If you have time to take several practice tests, take the first one open book, with no time limit. Work through the questions at your own pace and make sure you fully understand them. Gradually work up to taking a test under test conditions: sit at a desk with all study materials put away and set a timer. Pace yourself to make sure you finish the test with time to spare and go back to check your answers if you have time.

After each test, check your answers. On the questions you missed, be sure you understand why you missed them. Did you misread the question (tests can use tricky wording)? Did you forget the information? Or was it something you hadn't learned? Go back and study any shaky areas that the practice tests reveal.

Taking these tests not only helps with your grade, but also aids in combating test anxiety. If you're already used to the test conditions, you're less likely to worry about it, and working through tests until you're scoring well gives you a confidence boost. Go through the practice tests until you feel comfortable, and then you can go into the test knowing that you're ready for it.

Test Tips

On test day, you should be confident, knowing that you've prepared well and are ready to answer the questions. But aside from preparation, there are several test day strategies you can employ to maximize your performance.

First, as stated before, get a good night's sleep the night before the test (and for several nights before that, if possible). Go into the test with a fresh, alert mind rather than staying up late to study.

Try not to change too much about your normal routine on the day of the test. It's important to eat a nutritious breakfast, but if you normally don't eat breakfast at all, consider eating just a protein bar. If you're a coffee drinker, go ahead and have your normal coffee. Just make sure you time it so that the caffeine doesn't wear off right in the middle of your test. Avoid sugary beverages, and drink enough water to stay hydrated but not so much that you need a restroom break 10 minutes into the test. If your test isn't first thing in the morning, consider going for a walk or doing a light workout before the test to get your blood flowing.

Allow yourself enough time to get ready, and leave for the test with plenty of time to spare so you won't have the anxiety of scrambling to arrive in time. Another reason to be early is to select a good seat. It's helpful to sit away from doors and windows, which can be distracting. Find a good seat, get out your supplies, and settle your mind before the test begins.

When the test begins, start by going over the instructions carefully, even if you already know what to expect. Make sure you avoid any careless mistakes by following the directions.

Then begin working through the questions, pacing yourself as you've practiced. If you're not sure on an answer, don't spend too much time on it, and don't let it shake your confidence. Either skip it and come back later, or eliminate as many wrong answers as possible and guess among the remaining ones. Don't dwell on these questions as you continue—put them out of your mind and focus on what lies ahead.

Be sure to read all of the answer choices, even if you're sure the first one is the right answer. Sometimes you'll find a better one if you keep reading. But don't second-guess yourself if you do immediately know the answer. Your gut instinct is usually right. Don't let test anxiety rob you of the information you know.

If you have time at the end of the test (and if the test format allows), go back and review your answers. Be cautious about changing any, since your first instinct tends to be correct, but make sure you didn't misread any of the questions or accidentally mark the wrong answer choice. Look over any you skipped and make an educated guess.

At the end, leave the test feeling confident. You've done your best, so don't waste time worrying about your performance or wishing you could change anything. Instead, celebrate the successful completion of this test. And finally, use this test to learn how to deal with anxiety even better next time.

Review Video: 5 Tips to Beat Test Anxiety
Visit mometrix.com/academy and enter code: 570656

Important Qualification

Not all anxiety is created equal. If your test anxiety is causing major issues in your life beyond the classroom or testing center, or if you are experiencing troubling physical symptoms related to your anxiety, it may be a sign of a serious physiological or psychological condition. If this sounds like your situation, we strongly encourage you to seek professional help.

Thank You

We at Mometrix would like to extend our heartfelt thanks to you, our friend and patron, for allowing us to play a part in your journey. It is a privilege to serve people from all walks of life who are unified in their commitment to building the best future they can for themselves.

The preparation you devote to these important testing milestones may be the most valuable educational opportunity you have for making a real difference in your life. We encourage you to put your heart into it—that feeling of succeeding, overcoming, and yes, conquering will be well worth the hours you've invested.

We want to hear your story, your struggles and your successes, and if you see any opportunities for us to improve our materials so we can help others even more effectively in the future, please share that with us as well. **The team at Mometrix would be absolutely thrilled to hear from you!** So please, send us an email (support@mometrix.com) and let's stay in touch.

> **If you'd like some additional help, check out these other resources we offer for your exam:**
> **http://mometrixflashcards.com/PainManagement**

Additional Bonus Material

Due to our efforts to try to keep this book to a manageable length, we've created a link that will give you access to all of your additional bonus material.

> **Please visit**
> **https://www.mometrix.com/bonus948/painmannurse** to
> **access the information.**